LIZ EARLE'S

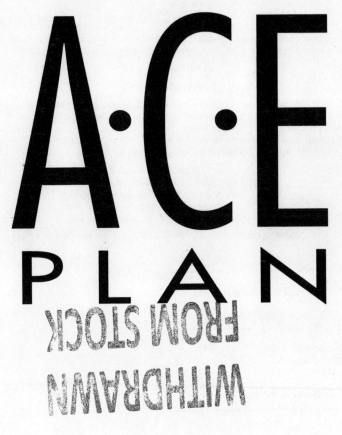

A·C·E

PLAN

First published in Great Britain in 1993 by Boxtree Limited,
Broadwall House, 21 Broadwall, London SE1 9PL

10 9 8 7 6 5 4 3 2 1

ISBN: 1 85283 518 4

Cover designed by Design 23
Illustrations by Raymond Turvey
Typeset by SX Composing Ltd, Rayleigh, Essex
Printed in Great Britain by
Whitstable Litho Printers Ltd., Whitstable, Kent.

A CIP catalogue entry for this book is available from the British Library

"Like small tremors before an earthquake, new studies on the role of vitamins are gently shifting the foundations of nutrition research, policy and public health."

Medical World News, Jan. 1993, Vol. 34, No. 1

CONTENTS

Acknowledgements

The research into antioxidants and free radicals is at the cutting-edge of biochemistry and I am grateful to the many senior scientists world-wide who have given information for this book. I am especially grateful to those I interviewed, including Professor Anthony Diplock and Dr Catherine Rice-Evans of Guy's Medical School, London, Dr Ruth Ames of UC Berkeley, Professor Charles Hennekens of Harvard Medical School, Professor Jeffrey Blumberg of Tufts University and Professor William Pryor of Louisiana State University. Also to Dr Stanley Rom, paediatrician at the Portland Hospital, London, for important help regarding infant feeding.

My thanks to Valerie Holmes of the Vitamin E Information Service for the excellent updates on an increasingly exciting and complicated subject. Also to Anne Moore and Michael Gordon for their support and information on beta-carotene. I am particularly grateful for the work carried out by my researchers Philippa McKinley and Annie Bawtree. A special word of thanks is also due to nutrition consultant Dr Derek Shrimpton for his careful editing and technical input.

Finally, I am grateful to my agent Rosemary Sandberg and publisher Michael Alcock for their support and encouragement, as well as to Wanda Whiteley and David Inman of Boxtree for their practical help. I also greatly value the unfailing enthusiasm and support I have received from Claire Bowles. On a practical note, I am indebted to my brother-in-law Brian Earle for the very necessary loan of his computer when my own Tandon failed at a critical time of writing. Also to my mother, Ann, Laura Hill and

Michelle McCarthy for feeding baby Guy during the nights! Last, but not least, I thank my husband Patrick for listening to my endless talk of free radicals and the all-important ACE vitamins.

Note: Nutritional references taken from McCance and Widdowson, *The Composition of Foods*, 5th edition. Royal Society of Chemistry, Ministry of Agriculture, Fisheries and Food.

INTRODUCTION

The Art of Healthy Living

The contents of this book will revolutionize the way we view food and vitamin supplements. Its implications for better health are enormous and far-reaching, and the theory behind it is backed by world-wide research at the highest levels.

What is the ACE Plan?

The Ace Plan is different from all other diet and lifestyle books as it offers every reader the chance to achieve a longer, healthier life.

How does it work?

The ACE Plan works by giving you the nutritional know-how to watch what you eat and put the latest scientific and medical findings into practice every day. Unlike any other eating plan, it does not insist on rigid rules or calorie-counted food. It is not about weight loss, but about health gain. Follow the advice given on all aspects of your lifestyle and you will feel fitter and younger for it.

What makes the ACE Plan so different?

The ACE Plan identifies a group of super-nutrients that are currently attracting the attention of both the medical and scientific worlds. In essence, these are the precursor to vitamin A (called beta-carotene), vitamin C and vitamin E – referred to throughout this book as the ACE vitamins. Together, these nutrients form a powerful alliance that can help protect the body from many of the diseases associated with growing old.

Where can I find the ACE vitamins?

You will find beta-carotene, vitamin C and vitamin E in everyday foods such as fruits and vegetables and cooking oils. They are also widely available in capsule and tablet form. It is not hard to find the ACE vitamins – the key is knowing where they are and making sure that we eat them in the right quantities.

How can the ACE vitamins help me?

In the last few years, medical research has moved away from concentrating on infectious diseases, which are now largely controlled by improved hygiene conditions. Today, most health problems are caused by degenerative disease created over time inside the body. The super-vitamins identified by the ACE Plan have the potential to protect every one of us against many diseases from within. The ACE vitamins can improve our quality of life at every age and may even slow down the ageing process itself. Not only do they improve our well-being, they also protect every single cell in our body. Top-level research around the globe shows that in combination, these vitamins are so powerful that they provide us with the potential to boost our immunity to life-threatening illness such as heart disease and cancer, prevent serious disorders such as cataracts and even reduce signs of ageing such as facial lines and wrinkles.

Prove it!

Researchers at the most highly respected medical and scientific centres around the world, including the Harvard Medical School in America, Oxford University and Guy's Medical School, London, are producing evidence to suggest that living longer and looker younger is as easy as learning your ACE. The ACE Plan reveals the research that is exciting nutritionists, doctors and scientists around the world. This book explains how you can achieve miraculous effects not only for yourself, but also for every member of your family. We need the ACE vitamins from the very moment we are born, right through until old age. Young and old alike will benefit from the very latest knowledge and enjoy the chance of better health that these nutrients offer.

1000 times safer than drugs

The ACE vitamins are present in many types of food and occur in our diet naturally. They have played an important part in mankind's development for thousands of years and are safe substances to take in the normal amounts available to maintain and encourage better health. Unfortunately, the same cannot be said of many of the prescription drugs used to treat degenerative diseases, and there is increasing concern over the use and efficacy of many of our common modern-day drugs. All drugs have side-effects but, more importantly, research is revealing that many of the so-called 'wonder drugs' simply do not live up to their original promise.

Yet the appalling rise in serious diseases, such as cancer, must be controlled, so what are the alternatives? We have known for many years that vitamins are vital for keeping us alive, and so it is no surprise that science should now turn its attention to vitamins' action against disease, in particular serious disorders such as heart disease and cancer. Studies show that vitamins and the use of supplements are 1000 times safer than drugs. In a five-year period, the only fatality due to taking vitamin supplements reported by American poison control centres was later found to be the result of an error. By contrast, during the same period, drugs of all kinds caused over 1000 deaths. (This does not include the figures for suicide by overdose.) By contrast, the vitamins in our food and in supplement products have been shown to be both useful and safe when it comes to disease prevention.

Action behind the scenes

The ACE Plan encourages better health and a longer life,

but it is neither a magical elixir of youth nor some quack guide written by cranks. Instead, it is based on the extensive research that has been carried out by several independent organizations for more than a decade. This research continues to be backed at the very highest levels, including the Ministry of Agriculture, Food and Fisheries (MAFF), which is spending more than £3 million on studying the ACE vitamins, and the World Health Organization which has a budget of many millions.

What the experts say

Here's what the experts have to say about the ACE vitamins, the antioxidant nutrients:

'We are opening up a whole new frontier for vitamins.' – Professor Ishwarlal Jialal, University of Texas South-western Medical Centre, USA

'There's ample evidence that antioxidants can help prevent cancer and other diseases.' – Gladys Block, Professor of Public Health Nutrition, University of California, USA

'The antioxidant nutrients are considered to have important potential in the prevention of several human diseases, in particular cardiovascular disease and some forms of cancer . . . They are of huge significance and will assume an increasing role in preventative medicine.' – Professor Anthony Diplock, Head of Biochemistry, Guy's Hospital Medical School, University of London

Clinical studies

There have been several hundred studies into the extraordinary powers of beta-carotene, vitamin C and vitamin E, many of which we shall examine in more detail a little later. Meanwhile, here are just a few of the impressive results:

- *Lung cancer*
  A twenty-year study involving 4500 men in Finland concluded that those with the highest intake of beta-carotene, vitamin C and vitamin E had the lowest levels of lung cancer. Even among non-smokers, it was found

that when the men were divided into three groups with low, medium and high levels of these vitamins, those in the lowest group were at least *twice as likely* to develop lung cancer as those receiving the most antioxidant vitamins.

- *Longevity*
A ten-year study of 11,000 men and women at the University of California, Los Angeles, found that those who took large amounts of vitamin C every day had a 25 – 45 per cent lower death rate of heart disease and a 10 – 42 per cent reduced mortality from all cancers, compared to those who took a substantially lower intake.

- *Heart disease*
A study of 500 men in Scotland found that the higher the levels of beta-carotene, vitamin C and vitamin E in their bloodstream, the lower their risk of angina. The study concluded: 'Populations with a high incidence of coronary heart disease may benefit from eating diets rich in natural antioxidants, particularly vitamin E.'

- *Heart disease and strokes*
A major American study involving more than 87,000 nurses over an eight-year period found that those who ate more beta-carotene had 40 per cent fewer strokes and 22 per cent fewer heart attacks than those who received less. In the same study, taking vitamin E capsules was associated with a 36 per cent lower risk of heart attack.

The oxygen of life

Human beings need oxygen to survive. The body uses oxygen to derive energy from food to fuel body processes. Oxygen is moved around the body by the red-coloured particles of haemoglobin which contain iron, (this is why our blood is dark red). Thanks to haemoglobin, our blood can absorb fifty times more oxygen than water. Oxygen is carried in the bloodstream throughout the body to feed all our living cells. The process of converting oxygen into energy is called *oxidation* and is essential for life.

This life-giving energy does, however, have a serious

side-effect, as oxygen also creates *free radicals*. Free radicals are constantly being created within the body: while you are reading these words they are being mass-produced inside you. Although a certain amount of free radical activity is needed by the body to kill bacteria, an excess quickly causes problems. If we make too many of them, however, they can cause many life-threatening illnesses. So although we need oxygen, it is a two-edged sword: on one side it gives us the breath of life we need to stay alive, but on the other it creates a damaging excess of free radicals that can lead to disease and death.

What are free radicals?

The term 'free radicals' sounds rather like the name of a terrorist group, and in a sense, this is a pretty accurate description. When too many free radicals are let loose inside the body they terrorize our cells; interfering with normal cell activity and causing change and damage. Free radicals are capable of reacting with almost every molecule in the body, causing them to become damaged, and researchers have linked these lethal particles to just about every degenerative disease.

Free radicals are largely produced by active forms of oxygen, as a by-product of oxidation. When oxygen is used by the body it burns food to make energy. It also burns germs and toxic substances such as ozone and carbon monoxide. These small fires give off 'sparks', or highly active free radicals. These damage the delicate membrane that surrounds our cells, disturb chromosomes and genetic material and destroy valuable enzymes, causing a chain-reaction of damage throughout the body. Research suggests that free radicals are a major contributor towards at least fifty of our most prevalent diseases, including coronary heart disease, lung disease, certain cancers, cataracts, rheumatoid arthritis, Parkinson's disease and even the ageing process itself.

The antioxidant answer

Antioxidants are the weapon we can use to fight the war

against excess free radicals, neutralizing them and preventing them from causing more damage within the body. Antioxidants have the ability to transform free radicals into less dangerous substances. Studies that look at how our bodies protect themselves from free radicals are often based on large population groups and have shown beyond doubt that low levels of the important ACE vitamins lead to high levels of disease.

How can we protect ourselves?

There are two ways in which we can reduce the damage caused by free radicals.

- First, we should avoid factors which encourage the production of free radicals. These include substances such as cigarette smoke, pollution and ultra-violet radiation from the sun, and we will take a closer look at these in the following chapter.
- The second course of action is to make sure we receive plenty of antioxidants in our daily diet. These include the all-important nutrients beta-carotene, vitamin C and vitamin E, which we will examine in detail in Chapter 2.

1

HOW TO LIVE LONGER

'It's not the years in your life, but the life in your years.'

Anon

The elusive elixir of life was long sought by the alchemists of the Middle Ages, and we are still waiting for its discovery! Biochemistry has now emerged as a science of the future which may hold the key to mankind's very survival. The research that is being carried out in laboratories around the world is unravelling many of the mysteries to do with disease and ageing. The question of whether the ACE vitamins actually add years to our lives may still be a matter for scientific debate, but these vital nutrients certainly seem able to increase our quality of life. After all, who wants to live to be 100 if this means being crippled with pain and mentally weak? The opportunity to lead a healthy, vigorous existence right up until the end is a much more attractive proposition.

In recent years, a few simple molecules, beta-carotene, vitamin C and vitamin E, have been causing quite a stir in the world of science and medicine. Collectively known as the antioxidant nutrients, they have the potential to keep us healthier and younger for longer.

The Free Radical Factor

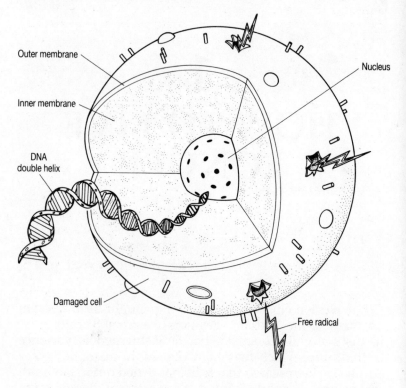

Outer membrane

Inner membrane

DNA
double helix

Damaged cell

Nucleus

Free radical

The enemy within

The antioxidant vitamins work by waging war on the invisible enemies inside the body. Beta-carotene, vitamin C and vitamin E are all engaged in the battle against excess free radicals as they are formed. The most effective strategy in any military campaign is 'know the enemy' and the same is true if we are to win the fight to remain fit and healthy. So the first step is to find out more about how and why free radicals occur.

One of our electrons is missing . . .

Free radicals are some of our foremost foes in the ageing process. To fully appreciate the damage they cause it is worth taking a quick chemistry lesson: 'Free radicals are molecular fragments with an unpaired electron.' Unfortunately, electrons are friendly creatures and prefer to go around in pairs. So they try to 'grab' another electron from a passing molecule to even themselves up. A free radical is a loose-living electron playing the field for a mate to settle down with. It will break up other pairs to find a partner and creates many more unstable molecules in the process. In short, a chain reaction occurs within the body which damages our cells.

As we saw in the Introduction, free radicals are continuously produced as a by-product of breathing in oxygen. Not all free radicals are damaging and a few are useful in helping our immune system. Some enzymes in the body need free radicals to work properly and they are also needed to expand our blood vessels and keep blood flowing freely around the body. Free radicals are also required to kill germs and help the white blood cells in our immune systems fight bacteria. This can be seen when we cut or graze our skin and a certain amount of inflammation appears before the wound heals. This reddish swelling is the action of free radicals attacking bacteria.

Problems arise when the body produces too many free radicals and the process gets out of control. It is the balance of free radicals, rather than the particles themselves, that is the key factor. Excessive numbers of free radicals end up damaging cell walls, destroying the genetic code called DNA that lives inside our cells, and causing the protein that holds our body together to disintegrate. This is pretty serious stuff. Although we are not aware of it happening at the time, the effects of this wholesale destruction of our cells is linked to just about every serious disease in the body.

DNA: What it means

- All life on earth, from grass to gorillas, is built around the genetic information carried within DNA, which is quite simply the most important molecule in the world. The scientifically minded will know that its initials stand for Deoxyribo-Nucleic Acid. All the messages of heredity are carried within DNA, which ensures that generations of living things continue to grow as they always have done.

- Molecules of DNA are packed inside every cell. If all the DNA could be uncurled from each cell it would measure about 2 metres (6½ feet) in length. The messages that DNA carries are extremely complicated and

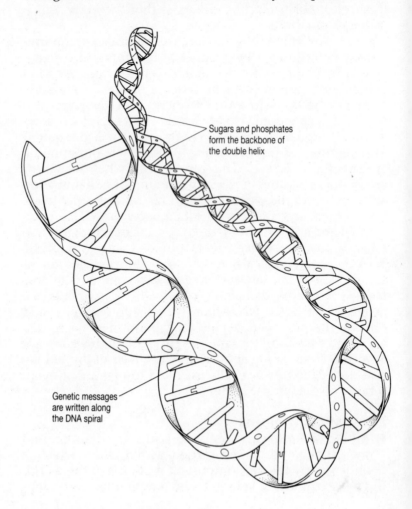

Sugars and phosphates form the backbone of the double helix

Genetic messages are written along the DNA spiral

human DNA contains enough information to fill over 1000 books the size of this one.

- DNA resembles two tiny chains twisted together to form a double helix or spiral. Genetic messages are written along these spirals in the form of chemicals known as 'base pairs'. These join the double helix together, like the steps on a spiral staircase. When cells divide and multiply, the double helix unzips and each side carries an identical set of genetic materials to two new cells.

- Free radicals damage DNA by attacking the sugars and phosphates that form the backbone of the double helix. Once these are damaged, DNA cannot give the correct instructions to make protein. This leads to mutations and substances which shouldn't be there being created inside the body.

How are free radicals formed?

Free radicals are produced by oxidation, the same process that causes butter to go rancid when it is left out of the fridge or cars to go rusty when exposed to the air. Although the body itself won't go rancid or rusty, its cells are affected in a similar way. This is why free radicals are so damaging. They are continually being produced in the body as an important component of our normal metabolism. In an ideal world, free radicals are dealt with by built-in safety mechanisms inside us, but they are also created by a number of outside influences, such as pollution, which is dramatically spreading in our environment. Our increasing exposure to factors such as pesticides, tobacco smoke, car exhaust fumes and ultra-violet radiation from the sun all add up to more free radicals being created than the body was originally designed to cope with.

How do free radicals damage us?

Excess generation of free radicals affect the body at its most basic level. They attack and infiltrate every living cell inside us. The prime targets of free radicals are the fats or lipids that make up our cell walls. Scientists refer to all kinds of fats as lipids and this type of attack is called lipid peroxidation, meaning that the fats around our cells have been altered by oxidation. One of Britain's leading experts on free radicals, Dr Catherine Rice-Evans, director of the Free Radical Research Group based at Guy's Medical School in London, explains:

'Inside the cell walls are various components that are doing different set tasks within the body. Free radicals attack the lipids and damage the cell membrane, causing these components to leak out. You can compare this to an egg with a damaged or broken shell – its contents leak out and make a mess. These components of the cell usually behave very well when they are inside their membrane, but when they escape and get to be somewhere they shouldn't, they becoming damaging. The important point about free radicals is the consequence of events that they cause – a destructive chain reaction.'

The chain reaction of free radical damage is also responsible for the premature death of a cell or the alteration of its response to hormones and neurotransmitters, signals from the brain. Free radical damage also prevents enzymes from regulating all bodily reactions and can even cause the mutations of our cells that lead to cancer.

More free radicals than ever

High levels of free radicals are commonly due to the increasing levels of pollutants in the atmosphere. We now breathe in more pollution in our air than ever before. We are also faced with a dramatically decreasing ozone layer which normally protects us from the free radicals that are formed by sunlight. Many health organizations have expressed concern over the rising levels of free radical damage. The Ministry of Agriculture, Fisheries and Food is certainly taking the issue very seriously and is funding extensive projects at the Free Radical Research Unit at Guy's Medical School. One of the areas of this research is examining the levels of antioxidant ACE vitamins in everyday foods, and we will look more closely at this in Chapter 2. As Dr Rice-Evans says, 'in ten years' time everyone in the street will recognize the importance of antioxidants.'

How the ACE Plan Can Help You

Are *you* at risk?

Good health is important at any age and you are never too young (or too old) to start benefiting from the ACE Plan. From the age of two to ninety-two, its fundamentals can work for you. The first step is to find out what goes on in your own life that makes you more or less vulnerable to free radical attack. Although this science is still in its infancy, there are a number of known risk factors.

To find out about your own current risk from the invisible attacks made by free radicals, simply complete the quiz on the next few pages. You will find score sheets at the end of the book where each member of the family can write their own answers. The scoring is designed to show your personal free radical risk. Once you have read through each section and answered all the questions, turn to page 42 for the scoring.

Section 1: Pollution

1. Where do you live?
a) in a city   ☐
b) in a city suburb   ☐
c) in the countryside   ☐

2. How many of these industrial sites are near where you live or work?
a) industrial factory or smoke stack   ☐
b) chemical factory   ☐
c) incinerator   ☐
d) solid-fuel power station   ☐
e) mining works   ☐

---

3. How many of the following are within half a mile of where you live or work?
a) main road or motorway ☐
b) busy road or high street ☐
c) airport flight path ☐
d) bus depot ☐

4. How often do you drive in traffic?
a) at least twice a day ☐
b) at least once a day ☐
c) three or four times a week ☐
d) once or twice a week ☐
e) rarely ☐

5. Does your work bring you into contact with hazardous chemicals such as dry-cleaning solvents, paints, printing or photographic chemicals, formaldehyde, ammonia, wood preservatives, glues, industrial cleaning materials, etc.?
a) yes, regularly ☐
b) yes, occasionally ☐
c) no ☐

Poisoned by pollutants

When we breathe in polluted air or tobacco smoke we are inhaling one of the most potent sources of free radicals. Although we cannot always see or smell them, many noxious substances, including carbon monoxide, nitrogen dioxide and lead from car exhausts, pollute the air we breathe. This remains an on-going problem in the industrialized Western world. Over half the population of America and a large proportion of people in Europe are currently breathing in toxins at levels that far exceed US Environmental Protection Agency 'ambient air quality' standards. In addition to car fumes, we are surrounded by many other invisible poisons. These include industrial pollutants such as cadmium, mercury and lead that escape into the atmosphere from battery-manufacturing, mining, smelting, foundries and metal-working. Toxic hydrocarbons are also released by paint-spraying, dry-cleaning, printing, oil refining, plastics manufacturing and chemical plants.

Our exposure to pollution continues and ground-level ozone is a serious problem for many smog-filled cities. Although ozone protects the earth when it is high in the sky, ground-level ozone is poisonous if directly inhaled, being created by other poisons in the atmosphere, such as nitrogen oxide from car exhausts. When we breathe in ozone it causes eye, nose and throat irritation and damages the lungs. High levels of ozone in the atmosphere also trigger asthma attacks.

Our lungs are the first major tissues in the body that these airborne sources of free radicals encounter. Once inside the lungs, free radicals assault the enzymes that enable our lungs to expand and contract. Without this elasticity, we find it hard to breathe and are unable to take in all the oxygen we need. In smokers, this can be seen in the disease called emphysema. Lung tissue is particularly vulnerable because it comes into direct contact with noxious substances as they are breathed in, and the cell walls in our lungs are extremely thin and delicate. As well as targeting the fatty part of the cell membranes in our lungs, these inhaled pollutants damage the watery parts of the cell, destroy red blood cells and damage our immune system. Inhaled toxins are also especially damaging because they proceed straight from the lungs to the rest of the body without passing through the liver for detoxification.

Air-borne pollution is extremely hard to avoid and it is impractical to suggest that we all leave our homes and jobs in the cities or suburbs and move to a cleaner environment in the Outer Hebrides. Fortunately, the ACE vitamins offer us some useful protection from the effects of pollution. A study reported in the *American Journal of Clinical Nutrition* in 1991, for example, shows that vitamin E is helpful in protecting us against the effects of ozone in smog. This is particularly important for children, who have been shown to be especially at risk from long-term exposure to pollutants because they have a higher metabolic rate and breathe in more air than adults. It is therefore essential to make sure that children receive adequate supplies of the antioxidant vitamins in their diet.

Although the ACE vitamins help combat the effects of poison in the air, pollution will also reduce our supply of these important nutrients. Studies have shown that city dwellers who breathe in polluted air have lower levels of antioxidant vitamins. Beta-carotene, vitamin C and vitamin E are needed throughout the body for many functions, but when we breathe in polluted air they are used up in the battle to fight free radicals. This leaves the rest of the body short-changed and dangerously low in supplies. If we run out of ACE vitamins, free radicals take over and a state known as 'oxidative stress' occurs. This means that the free radicals have won the war and can go on to cause damage throughout the body.

Section 2: Smoking

6. Do you smoke?
a) yes ☐
b) no (proceed to question 3) ☐

7. How many cigarettes do you smoke?
a) at least twenty a day ☐
b) between ten and twenty a day ☐
c) between five and ten a day ☐
d) less than five a day ☐
e) less than five a week ☐
f) the odd cigarette on rare occasions ☐

8. How many smokers do you live with?
a) more than three ☐
b) more than two ☐
c) more than one ☐
d) one ☐
e) none ☐

9. How often are you with other smokers?
a) everyday at work and socially ☐
b) everyday at work only ☐
c) everyday socially ☐
d) occasionally someone smokes near me ☐
e) rarely does someone smoke near me ☐
f) I do not allow anyone to smoke near me ☐

Stub it out!

It has been estimated that in industrialized countries tobacco is now causing about 2 million deaths a year, killing at least a third of those who regularly smoke cigarettes. Smoking a cigarette is equivalent to force-feeding the body with free radicals. Cigarette, cigar and pipe smoke contains over forty known cancer-causing compounds, including carbon monoxide, hydrogen cyanide, nitrogen dioxide and cadmium. Smoking tobacco also causes an increase in our own inflammatory cells that are themselves potent producers of free radicals.

Steps to discourage smoking certainly save lives. Smokers are often defensive about their filthy habit and commonly complain of feeling persecuted, but according to Dr Richard Peto, consultant in infectious diseases at the John Radcliffe Infirmary in Oxford, 'The real defenders of smokers are those who provide clear and accurate information about the large risks, and the real persecutors are those in journalism or, particularly, in advertising who seek to obscure the medical evidence.'

Cigarette smokers may cite their right to smoke, but they have no right to poison the air. Smoking damages passive smokers as well as the addicts themselves. In fact, the burning end of a cigarette produces nitrogen dioxide, a powerful free radical, which is then inhaled by the non-smoker. This sidestream smoke is potentially even more dangerous than the mainstream smoke exhaled by the smoker. Studies have shown that the spouse of a heavy smoker is more than three times as likely to develop lung cancer than the spouse of a non-smoker. Children whose parents smoke are also particularly at risk, as the free radicals they breathe in damage their developing tissues. Dr William Cahan, a specialist in lung cancer at the Memorial Sloan-Kettering Cancer Centre in America, bluntly states that 'Parents who smoke in the presence of their children are committing child abuse.'

According to Professor Nicholas Wald of St Bartholomew's Hospital, London, passive smoking increases children's risk of pneumonia and glue-ear – the most common cause of deafness in children – by about 50 per cent. Smoking during pregnancy will harm a baby in the womb and the risks continue after birth, with smoking linked to low birth weight, cot death, bronchial damage and childhood asthma. It may also affect a child's mental development later on. Smokers who breast-feed should also be aware that they are passing toxic chemicals on to their babies.

Action for passive smokers

It seems there is no end to the long list of damage caused by cigarette smoking, not only for the smokers themselves, but also for those who breathe in the smoke from others.

There is increasing evidence that smokers and passive smokers need higher levels of ACE vitamins in their diet, in particular to combat the damage being done to their lungs.

Cigarette smokers have lower levels of vitamin C in their bloodstream than non-smokers: in a recent American study, it was found that smokers needed to consume at least 150 mg of vitamin C a day (the amount found in four fresh oranges) in order to achieve blood-levels of the vitamin comparable to those found in non-smokers. Other more conservative figures estimate that smokers need between 70 and 80 mg a day more than non-smokers.

Vitamin C is an important part of the collagen that keeps our complexion smooth, which may be one reason why studies at the Wilson Dermatology Clinic in North

Carolina have found that smokers have many more facial lines and wrinkles than non-smokers. Other studies show that levels of beta-carotene are also low in smokers. One survey found that those who smoked a packet of cigarettes a day had 25 per cent less beta-carotene in their blood than non-smokers, despite consuming the same amount in their food.

Section 3: Radiation

10. Do you live near an airport?
a) yes ☐
b) no ☐

11. Do you live within sight of overhead power lines?
a) yes ☐
b) no ☐

12. How much time do you spend each day in front of a TV or computer screen?
a) three hours or more ☐
b) two hours or more ☐
c) one hour or more ☐
d) less than one hour ☐
e) none ☐

13. How often do you use a microwave oven?
a) at least once a day ☐
b) at least once a week ☐
c) occasionally ☐
d) never ☐

14. How much time do you spend outdoors each day?
a) most of the day ☐
b) a few hours a day ☐
c) less than an hour a day ☐

---

15. During the summer months, how much time do you spend outdoors encouraging a sun tan?
a) I spend a lot of time building up a sun tan ☐
b) I spend a moderate amount of time in the sun ☐
c) a couple of hours a week are spent in the sun ☐
d) almost no time is spent in the sun ☐

16. How much time do you spend in hot climates abroad?
a) several months of the year ☐
b) at least one month a year ☐
c) an annual two-week holiday to the sun ☐
d) one week or less ☐
e) none ☐

17. When you are in the sun, do you use a sun-block to protect your skin?
a) yes, always ☐
b) yes, frequently ☐
c) yes, occasionally ☐
d) no, never ☐

Radiation risks

Radiation is a general term which refers to energy waves and there are many different bands within the spectrum. The wave-length determines the type of radiation, for example light waves, radio waves and microwaves. In terms of causing free radicals, the most potent forms of radiation come from nuclear energy, X-rays and sunlight. Television screens, VDUs and computers all produce electro-magnetic radiation, which creates static but has a less certain link with free radicals. However, there is some evidence to suggest that electro-magnetic radiation does encourage free radicals once they have formed, even though the subject of electro-magnetic radiation and free radicals is still very much a speculative area of research. Dr Keith McLauchlan, a leading researcher in the field of physical chemistry at Hertford College, Oxford, suggests that the possible link between electricity and cancer is due to free radicals, which his research has shown to respond to electro-magnetic fields such as those surrounding power-lines. These free radicals may be produced in greater quantity and encouraged to live slightly longer, thus increasing the chance that they will damage the DNA in our cells. So although it is not yet clear what long-term effect electro-magnetic radiation has on our health, it does encourage free radicals, and while this may not be obviously damaging, it is clearly undesirable.

Dying for a tan?

The sun's rays give us life, light and warmth. Unfortunately, however, this welcome sunlight also carries with it a dangerous form of ionizing radiation that generates free radicals. The sun emits waves of energy in the form of ultra-violet radiation: the two main wave-bands are called UVA and UVB. Even on a cloudy day we receive doses of both UVA and UVB radiation through our skin.

UVA makes up about 80 per cent of all the ultra-violet radiation we are exposed to. UVA rays not only hit the skin, they pass straight through the upper layers and reach the dermis below. Down in the dermis the UVA rays destroy the supporting collagen and elastin fibres of the skin as well as generating free radicals. UVA radiation is the main cause of premature skin-ageing as it produces wrinkles and a loss of firmness – although UVA sunbeds probably won't give you skin cancer, they will make your skin sag.

UVB rays account for about 20 per cent of the radiation we are exposed to. This wave-band is mainly absorbed in the upper level of the skin where it stimulates the production of the brown pigment called melanin which gives us our sun tan. Too much UVB radiation causes the skin to redden and burn. UVB rays also damage the DNA in cells and are the main cause of skin cancer as they generate large numbers of free radicals. A simple way to remember the effects of ultra-violet radiation on the skin is that UVA rays mainly cause AGEING, while UVB rays are largely responsible for BURNING.

Some types of skin cancer can be fatal. Malignant melanoma is the most serious form and is increasingly common. In fact, deaths due to skin cancer have been doubling every decade and this is largely due to the fact that we are receiving more UVB radiation from the sun. Dr Rice-Evans confirms that 'melanoma is a direct result of free radical action on the skin from a radiation source. Those most at risk have naturally pale skins, i.e. the North European races.'

Skin cancer risks
Cases of malignant melanoma are rising every year.

- In 1930 our risk was 1 in 1500

- In 1990 it had risen to 1 in 123

- In 2000 our estimated risk will be 1 in 90

There are two main reasons why the rate of skin cancer is rising so rapidly. First, we tend to spend more time in exotic holiday locations where the sunshine is stronger and more deadly. Second, the ozone layer that would normally shield us from the sun's rays overhead is being depleted at an alarming rate. There is now such a large hole in the ozone layer above Australia, for example, that two out of three Australians will have suffered some form of skin cancer by the age of seventy-five. Unfortunately, skin scientists are predicting similar problems for Britain because the ozone layer has also reduced by at least 8 per cent over Europe and it is estimated that by the year 2000 it will have reduced by 30 per cent. Any reduction in the ozone layer inevitably means more radiation on the ground below. In turn, this results in more free radicals being formed inside the body.

Section 4: Alcohol

18. Do you drink alcohol?
a) yes, often ☐
b) yes, occasionally ☐
c) no, never ☐

19. Do you drink more than the recommended daily allowance of 3 units of alcohol a day for men, 2 units a day for women? (Each unit is the equivalent of half a pint of beer or lager, a glass of wine, a single measure of spirit or a small glass of sherry.)
a) yes ☐
b) no ☐

20. Do you ever drink alone?
a) yes ☐
b) no ☐

21. Do you ever suffer from hangovers?
a) yes, often ☐
b) yes, occasionally ☐
c) no, never ☐

We all know by now that excessive drinking of alcohol is bad for us. Alcohol is not only a powerfully addictive drug, but too much also leads to large numbers of free radicals in the liver.

In the midst of all this bad news, however, it is cheering to learn that moderate amounts of alcohol may actually be good for us! Red wine in particular has been found to contain powerful antioxidant substances than can neutralize free radicals. These antioxidants come not from the alcohol itself, but from substances called *procyanadins*, found in grape skins. Procyanadins are found only in red wine because the vinification process involves the grape skins being left in contact with the wine. However, as almost all

grapes are heavily sprayed with fungicides which themselves produce free radicals in the body, the most sensible
answer may be to choose organic varieties of red wine
which have been produced without pesticides. As with all
things, though, moderation is the key.

In heavy drinkers, alcohol, as well as drugs such as
paracetamol, can interact with normal liver biochemistry
and produce free radicals which damage liver tissues. This
is believed to be the cause of cirrhosis of the liver and liver
failure. All dietary studies of heavy drinkers have also
found disturbingly low levels of vitamin C, thought to be
caused by bad eating habits and the direct effect of alcohol
preventing the metabolism of vitamin C.

Section 5: Diet

22. How often do you eat fried foods?
a) at least once a day ☐
b) two or three times a week ☐
c) once a week or less ☐
d) never ☐

23. How often do you eat salt-cured, salt-
pickled or smoked foods, for example,
meat products such as salami, smoked fish
etc.
a) at least once a day ☐
b) two or three times a week ☐
c) once a week or less ☐
d) never ☐

24. How often do you eat sausages or other
processed meat products?
a) at least once a day ☐
b) two or three times a week ☐
c) once a week or less ☐
d) never ☐

25. How often do you eat barbecued food?
a) at least once a day ☐
b) two or three times a week ☐
c) once a week or less ☐
d) never ☐

26. Do you buy organically grown fruits, vegetables and other produce?
a) yes, always ☐
b) frequently ☐
c) occasionally ☐
d) never ☐

27. How many portions of fruit and vegetables do you eat each day?
a) five or more ☐
b) four or more ☐
c) three or more ☐
d) two or more ☐
e) one ☐
f) none ☐

28. Do you eat at least two slices of wholemeal bread a day (or other wholegrain products such as wholewheat pasta or oatbran)?
a) yes ☐
b) no ☐

Free radicals in food

We are increasingly at risk from free radicals in our food. The main source is fats, such as cooking oils, when they are heated to high temperatures. As fats are heated, their chemical structure breaks down to form peroxides. These then break down further to form the dangerous hydroxyl radical. This type of free radical is highly reactive and causes a great deal of damage to our cells and DNA. Professor Diplock explains that 'when our DNA is attacked in this way it causes mutagenesis which may then go on to cause cancer'. The occasional fry-up won't kill us, of course, but eating fried foods regularly over twenty or thirty years may well build up enough altered and toxic products within the body to affect our basic biochemistry and lead to disease.

Polyunsaturated fats such as sunflower and safflower oil are the least stable at high temperatures. These become 'oxidised' more quickly than monounsaturated fats, such as olive oil. The best option when frying foods, therefore, is to use olive oil. Dr Rice-Evans explains that 'an oil will oxidize if it has two or more double bonds in its chemical structure (such as polyunsaturated sunflower oils). As olive oil only has one double bond it is very much more stable when cooking. It is the only vegetable oil I use in my kitchen.'

The lipid peroxidation that occurs when heating a cooking oil can be prevented by vitamin E, in which vegetable oils are naturally rich, although its exact content depends on the extent the oil has been tampered with. Natural, unrefined corn oil, for example, has plenty of vitamin E to prevent peroxidation, but when it is refined and stripped of its natural constituents to produce a light, clear oil it loses at least a third of its vitamin E. In general, pale, clear cooking oils have the least vitamin E and are the most susceptible to peroxidation. The same is also true of low-fat spreads and margarines that are made from highly refined oils. Some manufacturers recognize this problem and are starting to put vitamin E back into their products, although unfortunately they often add synthetic vitamin E which is not as potent as the natural variety. The answer is to buy unrefined and cold-pressed oils which are likely to contain higher levels of vitamin E.

All oils need careful storage. Polyunsaturated oils such as sunflower and safflower are broken down by heat and light, so they are best kept in the fridge. Olive oil is more robust and may be kept at room temperature. It is important that all oils are stored in a dark place, as light will spoil an oil 1000 times faster than oxygen from the air. Because oils oxidize when exposed to the air, they should also be kept tightly sealed. Don't leave the top off the bottle for longer than necessary. It is better to buy cooking oils in small quantities and replace them frequently.

Tips for healthy frying

- Buy oils that have been packaged in dark glass containers or tins as these will have been better protected from the light.
- Buy darker cooking oils, such as olive oil, or unrefined sunflower oil (available from health food shops). These oils contain higher levels of natural vitamin E than the pale, highly refined and deodorized oils.
- Heat the frying pan *before* pouring in the oil to preserve its chemical structure for longer.
- Use a non-stick frying pan which requires only minimal oil.
- Never re-use cooking oil. It loses its vitamin E after heating and repeated cooking creates more toxic peroxides.
- When frying vegetables, add a little water to the oil. This helps keep the temperature down, produces steam to protect the oil from the air, and speeds up cooking time.
- Choose a monounsaturated oil such as olive oil or sesame seed oil for frying.
- Store all oils in a cook, dark place.

Altered food states

Although monounsaturated vegetable oils, such as olive oil, are believed to be healthy, some oils can pose a problem when they are processed. Trans-fatty acids are artificially created in food processing when fats are chemically altered from the natural *cis*-form of fatty acids. Trans-fatty acids are principally produced during the process of hydrogenation, whereby a liquid vegetable oil is hardened through the use of hydrogen gas to make a solid fat. Hydrogenation allows a cheap cooking oil to be turned into a semi-solid or hard fat with a long shelf-life. These fats are primarily found in margarines and low-fat spreads, and are also widely used in making cakes, biscuits, crackers and many other processed foods.

The process of hydrogenation and the creation of trans-fats have worried some nutrition researchers for a number of years. The hydrogenation process is a special cause for concern as it has been linked to heart disease. A recent study carried out by researchers at the Harvard Medical School in Boston and published in the medical journal *The Lancet*, connects trans-fatty acids to an increase in coronary heart disease. The study involved 85,000 women over a five-year period: when their intake of trans-fatty acids was analysed, there emerged a clear relationship between high levels of these fats and high rates of heart disease.

Free radicals are also created by several food processes. Many foods, such as darkly browned toast and barbecued meats, are burned in the cooking process. This burning is caused by the production of large numbers of free radicals. The long-term implications are unknown, and the odd piece of charred toast is unlikely to do much harm, but burnt foods should not be eaten too often. Charred foods, especially fatty foods, such as barbecued sausages, also contain a higher concentration of cancer-causing substances and are best avoided. Salt-cured and salt-pickled foods have also been linked to cancer as some contain nitrite. This substance is acted upon by free radicals to create nitrosamines which are some of the most carcinogenic substances known to man. Fortunately, the formation of nitrosamines is prevented by the antioxidant nutrients, including vitamin C and vitamin E.

These antioxidants are also added to many foods to act as natural preservatives. For example, vitamin E is added to some fats and oils to delay rancidity and vitamin C is used as an 'improver' to make the gluten in white bread more elastic, which produces a softer loaf. Antioxidants added to foods can be identified on food labels as follows:

- Vitamin E is listed as E306-E309. Natural Vitamin E is listed as E306. E307 – E309 are all synthetic forms of vitamin E.

- Vitamin C is listed as E300-E304. It may also be called l-ascorbic acid.

Although levels of added nitrites in food are low, high levels of other nitrates in our drinking water cause a problem. Nitrates can turn into nitrites in the presence of certain bacteria and fungi and this has been shown to be strongly linked to cancer. In recent years the levels of nitrates in our drinking water have greatly increased. This is because they are added to soil in the form of fertilizers where they leach out into rivers and streams to end up in our tap water. The EC limit for nitrate in drinking water is fifty parts per million (ppm), although for many years several water authorities have exceeded this. Some types of water filter will reduce the levels of nitrates in tap water, or alternatively you can buy bottled water that specifies a low nitrate level. This precaution also reduces other sources of free radical activity in our water supply, such as chlorine and some pesticides.

Section 6: Exercise

29. How often do you take some form of vigorous, aerobic exercise (any exercise or sport that makes you short of breath)?
a) every day ☐
b) two or three times a week ☐
c) once a week ☐
d) rarely ☐
e) never ☐

30. How much time do you spend taking some gentle form of exercise (including walking the dog, housework, gardening, etc.)
a) two or more hours a day ☐
b) one or more hours a day ☐
c) less than one hour a day ☐
d) none ☐

---

31. How often do you play sport?
a) every day ☐
b) two or three times a week ☐
c) once a week ☐
d) rarely ☐
e) never ☐

Exercise and free radicals

There is no doubt that we all benefit from taking plenty of exercise, but even this healthy pursuit has its downside. All those who exercise regularly, whether they are world-class athletes or uncompetitive joggers, breathe in much more air while working out – this ranges from ten to twenty times more than average for a well-trained athlete. Unfortunately, more oxygen within the system means more free radicals being produced. Excessive rates of oxygen consumption can cause damage to cells during and after exercise, making the muscles more susceptible to injury. In the case of professional athletes, it has been found that many of those who have over-training complaints such as torn ligaments, aches and strains, have evidence of oxidative damage in their tissues. This is because when a sports injury occurs the immune system is called into action to remove damaged cells. Two particular parts of the immune system called *monocytes* and *neutrophils* do the clean-up job, but they release free radicals in the process and are often over-enthusiastic in their task, resulting in pain, swelling and inflammation.

We must also guard against exercising outdoors when the air quality is poor. All forms of exercise require us to breathe in more deeply and we end up absorbing greater quantities of pollutants this way. Trials with top-class athletes, including those who train outdoors, show they have lower levels of vitamin E in their blood plasma and red blood cells. This is probably because their bodies are using vitamin E to fight the extra free radicals created by exercise. Researchers at Tufts University in Boston suggest that one answer may be to supplement exercise routines with a daily dose of ACE vitamins. Studies show that vitamin E in particular reduces tissue damage and helps muscles to recover and regenerate more quickly after exercise.

Anyhow, there is certainly no excuse for us all to become couch-potatoes overnight! Exercising is extremely good for the body as a whole because it offers many other health benefits, such as lowering blood pressure, stimulating the circulation, reducing signs of stress and preventing excessive weight gain. Clearly, we must continue with our exercise regimes, even if this only involves taking the dog for a daily run.

Section 7: Genetics

32. Have any of your close family members had any form of heart disease?
a) yes, one or both parents ☐
b) yes, a distant relative ☐
c) no ☐

33. Have any of your close family members suffered from cancer?
a) yes, one or both parents ☐
b) yes, a distant relative ☐
c) no ☐

34. Have either of your parents died from a disease before the age of seventy-five?
a) yes, both parents ☐
b) yes, one parent ☐
c) no, both parents are under the age of seventy-five ☐
d) no, both parents are over the age of seventy-five ☐

Heredity plays an important part in many diseases and it has been said that we should all choose our parents carefully! The genetic material that we inherit from our parents is an integral part of all our cells and clearly influences our pattern of health. Obviously, we can't alter our genetic make up, but we do have the opportunity to protect ourselves from diseases to which we know we might be susceptible. For example, if there is a history of heart disease in your family it is prudent to avoid smoking, cut down on the amount of saturated fat you eat and increase your intake of vitamin E. Likewise, if there have been cases of certain cancers in your family, eating plenty of foods rich in beta-carotene is a wise idea (see page 52).

Scoring

Section 1: Pollution

Q.1	a	3
	b	2
	c	1
Q.2	score 1 point for each answer	
Q.3	score 1 point for each answer	
Q.4	a	5
	b	4
	c	3
	d	2
	e	1
Q.5	a	5
	b	3
	c	0

Section 2: Smoking

Q.6	a	5
	b	0
Q.7	a	6
	b	5
	c	4
	d	3
	e	2
	f	1
Q.8	a	4
	b	3
	c	2
	d	1
	e	0
Q.9	a	5
	b	4
	c	3
	d	2
	e	1
	f	0

Section 3 Radiation

Q.10	a	5
	b	0
Q.11	a	3
	b	0
Q.12	a	4
	b	3
	c	2
	d	1
	e	0
Q.13	a	3
	b	2
	c	1
	d	0
Q.14	a	3
	b	2
	c	1
Q.15	a	6
	b	3
	c	2
	d	1
Q.16	a	4
	b	3
	c	2
	d	1
	e	0
Q.17	a	0
	b	1
	c	2
	d	3

Section 4 Alcohol

Q.18	a	2
	b	1
	c	0
Q.19	a	5
	b	0
Q.20	a	5
	b	0
Q.21	a	6
	b	3
	c	0

Section 5 Diet

Q.22	a	3
	b	2
	c	1
	d	0
Q.23	a	3
	b	2
	c	1
	d	0
Q.24	a	3
	b	2
	c	1
	d	0
Q.25	a	4
	b	3
	c	2
	d	0
Q.26	a	0
	b	1
	c	2
	d	3
Q.27	a	0
	b	1
	c	2
	d	3
	e	4
	f	15
Q.28	a	0
	b	2

Section 6 Exercise

This section has higher scoring for those who exercise more frequently as this increases free radical activity.

Q.29	a	5
	b	4
	c	3
	d	2
	e	1
Q.30	a	4
	b	3
	c	2
	d	1
Q.31	a	5
	b	4
	c	3
	d	2
	e	1

Section 7 Genetics

Q.32	a	5
	b	3
	c	0
Q.33	a	2
	b	1
	c	0
Q.34	a	5
	b	3
	c	0
	d	−9

What your score means

The minimum score is zero and the maximum is 150. Most of us will fall somewhere between the two. The higher your score, the more at risk you are from excess free radicals and low levels of the ACE vitamins.

0 – 30 Congratulations! You are probably fortunate enough to live in a clean environment with few pollutants to worry about. You may already be watching what you eat and drink to ensure your vitamin levels are kept high. Check your score to see in which sections you scored the most marks. This will reveal the areas of your lifestyle that will benefit most from following the ACE Plan.

31 – 50 Well done – you are already benefiting from a fairly healthy lifestyle. Keep up the good work, especially by adding fresh fruit and vegetables to your diet and watching your alcohol intake. Be aware of the factors that cause free radicals, such as pollution and smoking, and try to avoid your exposure to them. If you live in a city you should consider increasing your intake of the ACE vitamins on a daily basis.

51 – 90 Watch out! you are probably exposed to several risk factors such as smoking and pollution. You need to take a closer look at what you eat and increase your consumption of fresh fruits and vegetables. This will boost your levels of the ACE vitamins. You could also consider taking supplements of the antioxidant nutrients, such as beta-carotene, vitamin C and vitamin E.

91 – 150 This score is high and means that you are exposed to many factors that encourage free radical activity. In turn, this indicates that you also have low levels of the important ACE vitamins. You should take serious steps to minimize your exposure to pollutants around you, including hazards at work and cigarette smoke. You should also closely examine your diet, cut down on fatty, processed foods and increase the amounts of fresh fruits and vegetables you eat. Aim for at least five portions of fruit and vegetables each day to increase your levels of protective ACE vitamins. You should also seriously consider taking a daily supplement of antioxidant nutrients, such as beta-carotene, vitamin C and vitamin E.

2
THE ACE VITAMINS

Living a longer, healthier and more energetic life is the aim of the ACE Plan. As we have seen, there are several ways in which the body is harmed by free radicals. Fortunately research shows that their damaging effects are greatly reduced by a few simple nutrients.

What are vitamins?
Vitamins are a handful of essential substances that act in various ways to keep us alive. We cannot do without them and if we don't get enough we can become ill and even die of vitamin deficiency. As you now know, the most important antioxidant nutrients are beta-carotene, vitamin C and vitamin E. Other useful nutrients with antioxidant properties are the minerals selenium, copper, manganese and zinc. We will take a closer look at these a little later in this chapter.

Why are the ACE vitamins so important?
Beta-carotene, vitamin C and vitamin E are known in nutritional jargon as antioxidants and they fight against the process of oxidation that occurs inside the body, and scientists are now recognizing the importance of this when it comes to growing old and developing serious

diseases. We can see the results of oxidation all around us in everyday life. For example, if you slice up an apple and leave it for half an hour the inside quickly turns brown, because the apple is reacting with oxygen in the air. Similarly, a car chassis will rust when left outside for long periods of time because it is exposed to oxygen in the atmosphere. An identical process is taking place within our own bodies every second of our lives. Although we can't see what's going on, our body is literally 'rusting' from within, due to this continual process of oxidation and the action of free radicals.

How do vitamins help?

The ACE vitamins and minerals that help to keep us youthful, fit and healthy are nature's answer to the damage caused by oxidation. Each of these nutrients works in a slightly different way, but their overall effect is to mop up the free radicals as they form and prevent them from going on to do serious damage within the body. As free radicals are continually created, it is well worth maintaining high levels of each of these vital vitamins.

All about Beta-carotene

Beta-carotene works in two different ways. It is firstly converted into vitamin A by the body and the leftover functions as an antioxidant. It is important not to confuse beta-carotene with vitamin A as the two are separate substances.

Vitamin A was one of the earliest vitamins to be discovered. In fact, records show that it was used way back in the year 1500 BC by the Ancient Egyptians to treat eye disorders such as night blindness. A lack of vitamin A is still the number one cause of blindness in underdeveloped countries today. Vitamin A was officially identified in 1913 by American researchers and there are two main types. One is found in foods that come from animals, such as meat and milk, and this form is called retinol. The other versions of vitamin A are the carotenoids that are found in fruits and vegetables. There are around 600 of these, but the most important one is beta-carotene. The body is able to convert beta-carotene into vitamin A as it needs it, which explains why vegetarians get all the vitamin A they need without eating any animal produce.

Vitamin A is one of our most important vitamins as it is needed for growth and for keeping our body tissues healthy. One of its most important roles is to reinforce the protective envelope or membrane that surrounds all our cells. Vitamin A also protects our mucous membranes, for example, those around the eyes and mouth. It is essential for good eyesight, and an early warning of vitamin A deficiency is night blindness and dryness of the conjunctiva and cornea known to the medical word as xerophthalmia. Although not a common problem in Britain, it is the number one cause of blindness in undeveloped countries. Vitamin A is also especially important for our skin and helps prevent dryness and flaking.

Vitamin A is a fat-soluble nutrient and so is only found in the fatty parts of food. It is present in meat (especially liver, where the animal stores its supplies of vitamin A) and in dairy products such as milk, butter and cheese. Fish liver oils are the richest natural source of vitamin A, which is one reason why a daily spoonful of cod liver oil does the body so much good. As with other fat-soluble nutrients, if we eat too much vitamin A, it ends up being stored in the liver, which is why eating large quantities of this vitamin can cause liver damage and excessive amounts may be linked to birth defects. For this reason, pregnant women are advised by the Chief Medical Officer not to take more than 750 mcg (2250 IU) of vitamin A (retinol) a day and to avoid eating liver more than once a week as it is such a rich source. Although large quantities of vitamin A can be toxic, the equivalent amount of its precursor, beta-carotene, is totally safe. Pregnant women who are concerned about their supplement intake could safely switch to beta-carotene instead. It is almost impossible to take too much beta-carotene as the body only converts it into the amount of vitamin A that it actually needs. Not only is beta-carotene non-toxic, it is also a powerful antioxidant and acts against free radicals. This makes it a preferable and altogether more exciting nutrient, for the reasons we shall now discover.

What is beta-carotene?

Beta-carotene is a natural plant dye and was first discovered in carrots, hence the name given to the entire family of carotenoids. The carotenoids are a colourful range of pigments which provide the huge variety of paintbox colours that we see in nature. Scientists first became interested in them over 150 years ago. In the 1830s researchers looking into the biology of plants pinpointed the yellow pigment that turns autumn leaves a different colour as being the carotenoid called lutein. Around fifty of the 600 carotenoids which have been identified since then can be converted by the body into vitamin A, but beta-carotene is by far the most effective. It is stored in the body in our fatty tissues and liver, and a small amount also circulates in the bloodstream.

Beta-carotene itself is a deep shade of red-orange and is the main pigment in yellow and orange fruits and vegetables. Foods rich in beta-carotene stand out on the supermarket shelves as they are brightly coloured, carrots and mangoes, for example. The riper the produce, the more beta-carotene it will contain. Dark green leafy vegetables such as spinach and broccoli also contain high levels of beta-carotene, although they are a different colour because the green chlorophyll pigment is more dominant. As a general rule, the darker and more vivid the colour of the fruit or vegetable, the more beta-carotene it contains. For example, dark Lollo Rosso lettuce leaves contain more beta-carotene than the pale iceberg variety.

In addition to the benefits of being converted into vitamin A as required, beta-carotene is now being studied the world over for another exciting property, namely as one of our most powerful antioxidants. The role of beta-carotene in plants is to help prevent fruits and vegetables from burning up in the sun. Free radicals are formed in plants (as well as in humans) by ultra-violet radiation from the sun, and so nature provides the antidote in the form of beta-carotene to ensure that the plants survive. Without protection from beta-carotene, our plant-life would be wiped out by the highly reactive singlet oxygen molecules created by the sun. It is not only plants that benefit from this parasol form of protection. Human beings also gain some sun protection from eating up their greens on a regular basis. Studies by Professor Micheline Matthews-Roth of the Harvard Medical School show that beta-carotene helps humans whose skin is overly sensitive to sunlight. Professor Matthews-Roth has spent over twenty years studying the effects of beta-carotene on the skin, and as a result the powerful US Food and Drug Administration (FDA) has approved it for the specific treatment of light-sensitive disorders. These are often a result of too many light-sensitive pigments being produced in the skin which encourage reactive singlet oxygen molecules. Beta-carotene helps by neutralizing the damaging effects of these molecules and calming the skin. Beta-carotene has also been tried out on other types of sun-sensitivity, such as prickly heat, and supplements for these disorders are available from a GP on prescription.

In addition to curing some skin disorders, beta-carotene may also protect normal skin from damage in strong sunlight. As we saw in the previous chapter, it is the tanning ultra-violet rays from the sun that also cause most of our wrinkles, and one way to help prevent this is to increase beta-carotene intake before setting off for the beach. Beta-carotene is also believed to help reduce the risk of sunburn, although we should always use high-protection sunscreens when our skin is exposed to strong sunshine. Although beta-carotene is non-toxic and safe to take in large quantities, it can have the peculiar side-effect of turning the skin orange! This is a result of the yellow/orange pigment temporarily staining the skin from within and can also happen if you regularly drink several cartons of carrot juice a day. Taking mega-doses of beta-carotene of around

300 mg daily can also cause temporary skin staining; indeed, many of the so-called 'suntanning pills' advertised are simply high-dose vitamin supplements, and if you really want to turn your skin an unusual shade of orange a cheaper option would be to swallow a handful of beta-carotene tablets.

Natural beta-carotene

There are two kinds of beta-carotene supplements, natural and synthetic. The natural beta-carotene pills are more expensive, and are much closer to the beta-carotene found in food. Man-made beta-carotene supplements come from petrochemicals and contain higher levels of trans-fats that make it more difficult for the body to use. Natural beta-carotene has lower levels of these unwanted trans-fats and is boosted by other members of the carotenoid family, such as lutein and alpha-carotene, which are also anti-oxidants. The natural beta-carotene found in supplements does not come from an obvious source, such as carrots, but from an unusual type of marine algae called *Dunaliella salina*. Algae, which have been around for millions of years and were among the earliest forms of life to appear on the planet, are extremely efficient at manufacturing beta-carotene to protect themselves from the sun's rays. *Dunaliella salina* grows in salt water in areas of the world where there is constant strong sunshine, such as Australia. It is harvested in nets so that the natural beta-carotene can be extracted and turned into capsules. When choosing a natural beta-carotene supplement, look for the words 'natural source' or 'natural *D.salina* beta-carotene' on the label.

The anti-cancer pill?

Apart from the welcome benefit of protecting the skin and discouraging wrinkles, the most important discovery concerning beta-carotene has been in the field of cancer. This disease currently kills more than 160,000 Britons every year and touches every family in the land since one in three of us are affected by cancer at some time in our lives and one in five people in Britain will die from it. While the medical world continues its search for elusive cancer cures, it seems that preventing the disease from happening in the first place may be a far easier option. Although no one knows exactly how or why cancer strikes, it is evident that those who eat the most beta-carotene also have the lowest rate of certain cancers. Numerous nutrition studies conducted on large populations have found that the risk of lung cancer and cancer of the stomach, oesophagus and cervix are all lower in those who eat plenty of beta-carotene. The same cannot be said of vitamin A, which suggests that it is the unusually powerful antioxidant quality of beta-carotene that has an anti-cancer action.

Scientists world-wide now believe that eating an abundance of fresh fruit and vegetables will provide sufficient beta-carotene to give significant protection against cancer. Although the existing evidence is limited, it has sparked major trials involving beta-carotene around the world. In America, 23,000 male doctors are currently taking beta-carotene supplements to see if the rate of cancer and heart disease can be lowered. In Finland, 19,000 smokers are being given daily doses of beta-carotene or vitamin E to see if either can prevent lung cancer. In China, where there is a high death rate from cancer of the oesophagus, those with pre-cancerous cell abnormalities are being given multi-vitamin supplements as part of their treatment. According to Dr John Bertram, director of basic science at the Cancer Research Centre of Hawaii, 'If these larger studies confirm the promise shown in earlier pilot studies, they will cause quite a revolution of thinking in this area.'

Beta-carotene may be especially successful at preventing cancer from occurring because it neutralizes the harmful effects of free radicals. When these destructive elements damage cells within the body, cancer is more likely to occur. Beta-carotene is clearly a powerful weapon as just one molecule of beta-carotene is able to mop up the energy of up to 1000 molecules of highly reactive singlet oxygen. There have been more than forty studies into the beneficial effects of beta-carotene on cancer, involving tens of thousands of people world-wide, and these will be explored further in Chapter 4.

How to measure beta-carotene

Beta-carotene is measured in micrograms (mcg or µg) and milligrams (mg). There are 1000 mcg to 1 mg. Some studies suggest we should be aiming for a minimum of 15,000 mcg (15 mg) a day. This level can only be achieved in our diet by eating *at least* five generous portions of fruits and vegetables every day. There's more about our daily vitamin needs in Chapter 5.

Where to find beta-carotene	
Food	**mcg per 100 g (4 oz)**
all vegetables are cooked unless otherwise stated; all fruits are raw	
carrots	4425
parsley (raw)	4040
sweet potatoes	3960
spinach	3840
watercress (raw)	2520
spring greens	2270
cantaloupe melon	1000
tomatoes	640
asparagus	530
broccoli	475
apricots	405
peaches	58

Cooking tips

Because beta-carotene is fat-soluble we absorb more from food if it is eaten at the same time as a little fat. For instance, dab a dot of butter on to cooked carrots or brush spring greens and sweet potatoes with a little olive oil.

Beta-carotene is relatively stable during food preparation and cooking, with only 15 per cent being lost when vegetables are cooked in a microwave oven. Processes such as blanching and freezing also have little effect on beta-carotene content (even tinned carrots have reasonable levels). However, over-cooking can decrease the amount of beta-carotene that is available for the body to use. Many vegetable sources, such as carrots, have hard cell walls which need to be broken down before the beta-carotene is released. For this reason, chopped, lightly cooked, and puréed vegetables such as carrots and spinach have a higher nutrient content. Vegetable juices, such as tomato, spinach and watercress, are excellent sources, too. Beta-carotene is also used by the food industry as a natural food colorant and crops up in many golden-yellow coloured foods, including butter, margarine and processed cheese.

Vitamin C

Vitamin C is probably the best-known of all vitamins, it is the one many of us turn to when attempting to ward off the common cold. Vitamin C has been shown to have many extraordinary properties, but the bottom line is that it is absolutely essential for keeping us alive. Without enough vitamin C in our diet we are at risk from infections and can even die from scurvy. Unlike other nutrients vitamin C has a strong social history as the result of this disease. In the seventeenth and eighteenth centuries scurvy was a common cause of death among sailors who lived at sea for months on end on a somewhat unbalanced diet of ship's biscuits and rum. It was not uncommon for a ship to lose more than half its crew to scurvy, just because of a lack of vitamin C. The symptoms of scurvy include swollen gums, loss of teeth and severe bruising under the skin. It is extremely painful and victims of this disease frequently died an unpleasant death. The link between vitamin C and scurvy was first investigated by a naval surgeon called James Lind. He was a Scotsman, born in 1716, and his family came from Dalry. By coincidence, Dalry is now the site of one of the largest vitamin C factories in the world, producing thousands of tonnes of the vitamin every year. When Lind was appointed ship's surgeon on HMS *Salisbury* he came across his first cases of scurvy and decided to test various cures. He found that the sailors who were given two oranges and a lemon recovered so quickly that they were soon able to resume their arduous duties. Unfortunately, his other patients who were fed a mixture of sea water, cider or vinegar did not do so well and usually died. Later, Captain James Cook arranged for supplies of concentrated lime juice rich in vitamin C to be distributed to his crew during long voyages at sea. This simple measure kept them alive and led to British sailors being known as 'limeys'.

Scurvy was not confined to the navy and has appeared throughout history at times of food shortages, such as during the sieges in the Middle Ages. It affected rich and poor alike, and some historians believe it killed King Henry VIII, who was notorious for his dislike of fruit and vegetables. Records show he lived almost entirely on meat and sugary puddings, and this lack of vitamin C could have been the cause of his swollen limbs, leg ulcers, blotchy skin and extreme irritability.

The introduction of the potato to Elizabethan England was a life-saver for many of the country's poor, who benefited most from this cheap, nutritious food. Indeed, vegetables were regarded as fit only for the working classes and, as a result, many of the aristocracy were affected by scurvy. Children were especially at risk during the late 1800s when it became fashionable to give up breast-feeding and wean children on to a diet of rusks and condensed milk. Many children died in appalling pain due to a simple lack of vitamin C in their diet. Those who survived were given simple doses of fresh orange juice.

Although it was recognized quite early on that citrus fruits could cure scurvy, the medical profession was at a loss to explain how. Animal experiments involving rats failed to show any connection, due to the fact that rats have the ability to make their own supplies of vitamin C, making it impossible for them to develop scurvy. It was not until scientists tried using guinea pigs in their dietary analysis that vitamin C was discovered, because the unfortunate guinea pig, like human beings, cannot manufacture its own supplies.

Chemically speaking, vitamin C is one of the simplest vitamins, which is why it was amongst the first to be studied. Yet, although it was officially identified over seventy years ago, scientists are still discovering fascinating new ways in which it works and this vitamin continues to excite nutrition researchers around the world. Its basic function is to help with the growth and repair of body tissues and to maintain healthy gums, blood vessels, bones and teeth. It is involved with the immune system and may also help the body fight off bacteria and viral infections. Vitamin C is mainly stored within the brain, the lungs and the adrenal glands which produce adrenalin. It is also essential to make collagen, the biological glue that sticks our cells together. Low levels of vitamin C in the body can lead to low levels of collagen, resulting in reduced elasticity of lung tissue which means that the lungs are not able to function properly. This is one plausible reason why elderly people with insufficient vitamin C intake are more likely to suffer from respiratory ailments such as bronchitis and pneumonia.

Vitamin C is also one of the antioxidant nutrients and so fights the formation of damaging free radicals. Unlike beta-carotene, vitamin C is water-soluble, and is therefore found in the fluids that flow between our cells. Vitamin C acts as a roaming soldier, fighting the free radicals that cross its path as it travels throughout the body. It is not stored in the system and so we need to eat foods that are rich in vitamin C every day to maintain a constant supply. It is impossible to take too much vitamin C as any excess simply passes through the body and is excreted in urine. The only side-effect of taking large quantities of vitamin C (upwards of 2000 mg or 2 g daily) might be mild diarrhoea, indeed high doses of vitamin C have even been used as a natural laxative!

Because vitamin C is metabolized using oxalic acid, a substance present in the formation of kidney stones, there has been a fear in the past that high doses of the vitamin could be a cause of kidney stones. However, there is no clear evidence of such a link, even with mega-doses of vitamin C, and it has been dismissed by researchers as a modern myth. Nevertheless, common-sense advice for anyone suffering from kidney problems is to avoid high doses of vitamin C which might raise oxalic acid levels.

Because it is an antioxidant, vitamin C acts as a natural food preservative by preventing the rancidity caused by free radicals. Also known as ascorbic acid, vitamin C is often used by the food industry as an additive to foods such as cakes and biscuits. Our best natural sources of vitamin C come from fruits and vegetables. For many years potatoes were its main source in Britain, but now that people tend to eat fewer potatoes, principal sources are fruit and fruit juices, especially orange juice. Raw foods, such as salads, are also a good source of vitamin C.

The bioflavanoids

In vitamin supplements, the natural form of vitamin C comes from acerola cherries or corn and is most effective when combined with bioflavanoids, a group of colouring pigments that top up plants' antioxidant protection against environmental stresses. Supplements that combine vitamin C with bioflavanoids are known as vitamin C Complex. Bioflavanoids are needed to strengthen the network of the capillary blood vessels that run throughout the body; they are especially important for the complexion and work in tandem with vitamin C to strengthen capillary walls and prevent bruising. All the fruits and vegetables that contain vitamin C are also a good source of bioflavanoids. These water-soluble nutrients occur in tiny quantities and cannot be stored by the body, which is why eating a regular supply of fresh foods is so important in order to maintain correct levels of vitamin C and bioflavanoids. A diet that is high in fresh fruit and vegetables typically provides a total of 1000-2000 mg (1-2 g) per day of the whole range of bioflavanoids. The best sources are the pith of citrus fruits, apricots, cherries, grapes, green peppers, tomatoes and broccoli.

Research into the bioflavanoids is in its infancy but is already turning up some interesting findings. For example, it is believed that by reinforcing cell membranes bioflavanoids may help prevent the leakage of excess antibodies into the bloodstream of allergy sufferers. This would make an allergic reaction less likely to occur and could spell relief for many millions of allergy sufferers. Certain bioflavanoids have also been found to block the production of inflammatory agents called leukotrienes in the body. As these are the foremost biochemical cause of asthmatic symptoms, the potential for using bioflavanoids to treat hay fever, asthma and other allergies is exciting.

Vitamin C and cancer

Studies have shown that people who eat more vitamin C have a reduced risk of cancer. About forty studies have been conducted on the relationship between vitamin C and cancer. According to Professor Gladys Block, nutrition specialist at the National Cancer Institute in America, the evidence for a protective effect of vitamin C against cancers of the oesophagus, larynx and oral cavity is 'strong and consistent'. There is also strong, although slightly less consistent, evidence that vitamin C protects against cancers of the cervix, colon, stomach and pancreas. In addition, a study by researchers at the University of California has found that those who consume high levels of vitamin C live longer generally and are particularly protected from heart disease. This is possibly because vitamin C works well with vitamin E, which has also been shown to help reduce the risk of heart disease.

How to measure vitamin C

Vitamin C is usually measured in milligrams (mg) or grams (g): 1000 mg is equal to 1 g of vitamin C. The recommended daily allowance (RDA) for adults in Britain is currently a mere 30 mg, although the new European recommendation is 60mg and many experts suggest that this should be raised to at least 100 mg. We will look at the reasons behind this move and discover our daily vitamin needs in Chapter 5.

Where to find vitamin C

all vegetables are cooked unless otherwise stated; all fruits are raw

Food	mg per 100 g (4 oz)
guavas	230
blackcurrants	200
parsley (raw)	190
green peppers (raw)	120
strawberries	77
kale	71
watercress (raw)	62
Brussels sprouts	60
lemons	58
oranges	54
broccoli	44
tomato purée	38
grapefruit	36
cauliflower	27
red cabbage	20
baked potatoes (with skin)	14
bananas	11
apples	6

Cooking tips

As vitamin C is destroyed by heat, the above foods are best eaten either raw or very lightly cooked. Of all the vitamins, it is vitamin C that disappears most quickly during cooking. This is because it is water-soluble and so dissolves into the cooking water. A good rule of thumb is to avoid using water to cook vegetables wherever possible. For example, a baked jacket potato eaten with the skin contains twice as much vitamin C as peeled, boiled potatoes: peeling vegetables before they are cooked results in a 10 per cent loss. Steaming vegetables or cooking them in the microwave are the best methods to preserve your vitamin C supplies. As much as 75 per cent of the vitamin C in green vegetables can be lost by simmering them in water, but if you do decide to cook them this way, vegetables such as cauliflower and broccoli are best placed directly into boiling water. This is because the oxidizing enzymes that destroy vitamin C do not work at high temperatures – they are most effective at around 60-85°C and so by putting vegetables into cold water and bringing them to the boil we destroy twice as many vitamins. Use a minimum of water as vegetables that are completely immersed lose up to 80 per cent of their vitamin C. If they are just one-quarter covered by water only about half as much vitamin C is lost. When cooking vegetables in water don't throw the vitamin C down the sink after draining but use the cooking water as a nutritious base for soup, sauce, stock or gravy. Cooking vegetables in a copper or iron pan should also be avoided as these metals react with vitamin C and destroy it.

Over-cooking is also a major cause of vitamin loss. Approximately 25 per cent of vitamin C is lost after 15 minutes' cooking time, rising to 75 per cent after 90 minutes. Vitamin C also escapes from food when it is exposed to the air, for example, after it has been cut, chopped or crushed. Food processing such as canning and bottling also affects the vitamin C content of foods, particularly fruits that contain dark red pigments. For example, strawberries can lose more than half their vitamin C when processed, and raspberries and blackcurrants even more. In addition, length of storage time also affects vitamin content. While freshly dug raw potatoes have around 30 mg of vitamin C per 100 g in October, this will have dropped dramatically to 8 mg by the following March. The key is to buy fresh fruit and vegetables when they are in season so you know they have not been sitting in cold storage for months on end. Once purchased, all fresh produce should be eaten quickly before it deteriorates further. This also applies to fruit juices: for example, apple juice loses half its vitamin C after four to eight days in the fridge; orange squash loses up to half its vitamin C content within a week of opening the bottle, and after three months it may have lost it all. Shaking the bottle or carton of juice lets more oxygen in and so destroys the vitamin C even faster.

Vitamin E

Vitamin E is possibly our most important free radical fighter because it protects every cell in the body. The term vitamin E was first used in 1922 to describe a substance discovered by scientists in vegetable oils that was essential to maintain fertility in rats: In 1936, an American research scientist, Dr Evans, isolated the most potent form of natural vitamin E from wheatgerm oil and analysed its chemical structure. He found that the term vitamin E actually applies to a whole family of chemical compounds called tocopherols, of which d-alpha tocopherol is the most effective. The technical name for vitamin E is *tocopherol*, which was used to describe the substance as it enabled the animals to have offspring. Tocopherol comes from the Greek *tokos* meaning 'birth' and *phero* meaning 'to bring forth'. Since its discovery, vitamin E has been nicknamed the 'virility vitamin' because it plays such an important part in human fertility. There is much more to vitamin E, however. This nutrient is essential for maintaining a healthy immune system as it strengthens white blood cells against infection and has particularly strong links with preventing heart disease. A study by the World Health Organization identified low levels of vitamin E as being the single most important risk factor in death from heart disease – more important even than high cholesterol, raised blood pressure or smoking. The other remarkable attributes of vitamin E include the ability to dissolve blood clots, strengthen blood capillary walls, improve the action of insulin in diabetics, increase muscle power and clean up pollution in our system. Vitamin E also influences hormonal processes, reduces the severity of inflammations and plays an important part in anti-ageing skin-care.

Too little vitamin E in the diet seriously impairs good health and leads to the loss of red blood cells, muscle wastage and sterility, although as is the case with vitamin C, a lack of vitamin E does not cause a clearly identified deficiency disease such as scurvy. The effects of eating too little vitamin E in our daily diet usually develop over long periods of time, and are linked with many degenerative disorders including premature ageing and arthritis.

Vitamin E is a fat-soluble vitamin and is therefore found in fatty tissues of the body including the protective membrane of all our cells. It is also found in the membrane that surrounds plant cells which is why we find small amounts in vegetables such as asparagus and spinach. In humans, vitamin E is stored in the areas of the body that need it most, including the heart, muscles, testes, uterus, blood, adrenal and pituitary glands. Extra supplies of vitamin E are also tucked away in the liver for future use; it is an extremely safe nutrient and it is virtually impossible to store too much of it.

Vitamin E as an antioxidant

Vitamin E is regarded as the single most important antioxidant nutrient. It works by preventing the oxidation or rancidity of fats, hence its especially important function in safeguarding the layer of protective fatty tissue which surrounds all our internal cells and major organs. Vitamin E is also an essential part of our daily diet as it prevents fats such as vegetable oils from turning rancid within the body. The more polyunsaturates we eat, such as those in sunflower oil spreads, the more vitamin E we need to consume. To neutralize free radicals as they are formed, vitamin E acts as a team with vitamin C. Once vitamin E has done its task of zapping a free radical, vitamin C re-activates it so that the molecules of vitamin E can carry on fighting. This is why it is so important to maintain adequate supplies of both vitamins C and E.

Natural vitamin E is best

The natural form of vitamin E that is found in foods is also the most effective in the body. Capsules and tablets of vitamin E containing natural vitamin E are made from vegetable oils, such as soya bean oil. Wheatgerm, sun-flower, corn, peanut and rapeseed oils may also be used and they all provide d-alpha tocopherol which is the single form of vitamin E. Synthetic vitamin E is made up of eight different substances, only one of which has the same molecules as natural vitamin E. The synthetic variety is produced from petrochemicals and is officially recognized as being 36 per cent less effective than natural vitamin E. However, recent studies indicate that natural vitamin E is more likely to be *twice* as effective than its synthetic counterpart. If you decide to take a supplement of vitamin E, do make sure it is the natural variety. Many brands now state that they contain natural source vitamin E. Alterna-tively, you can recognize the type of vitamin E by the wording on the label. The natural variety begins with the letter 'd', as in d-alpha tocopherol, and synthetic begins with a 'dl', as in dl-alpha tocopherol.

Vitamin E for a healthy heart

Vitamin E has hit the headlines with exciting research that shows we can lower our risk of heart disease with natural vitamin E supplements. The most recent data, published in the *New England Journal of Medicine* in June 1993, in-volved over 87,000 nurses. Harvard University researchers observed a protective effect in those taking a daily supple-ment of more than E 100 IU (international units) of vitamin E a day. This protection against heart disease was seen *only* in those women who were taking the supplement. No such results were observed in those who adjusted their diet to include more vitamin E-rich foods. Those who had taken vitamin E supplements for two or more years had half the risk of heart disease of those who had taken no supplement. This finding is extremely significant, and has resulted in greater studies currently being carried out to determine if we should all be taking a daily dose of vitamin E to maintain a healthy heart. Another study of almost 40,000 American male health professionals also supports a strong association between a high intake of vitamin E and a low risk from coronary heart disease. Interestingly, this time the researchers could not find such a link with vitamin C, and the benefits of beta-carotene were only found to be with smokers and former smokers. It may be that vitamin E is our most powerful antioxidant ally in the fight against heart disease.

How to measure vitamin E

Vitamin E should be measured in mgs, but international units (IU's) may be given for additional information. 1 mg of natural vitamin E (d-alpha-tocopherol) is equivalent to 1.49 IU (see the conversion table on page 164). At present, there is no recommended daily allowance (RDA) for vitamin E in Britain, although the European guidelines recommend 10 mg daily. Much of the recent research into vitamin E and disease prevention has involved larger doses. It is up to individuals to decide how much vitamin E to include in their diet and we will examine this issue further in Chapter 5.

Where to find vitamin E

Foods containing high levels of vitamin E are surprisingly scarce.

Food	mg of vitamin E per 100 g (4 oz)
wheatgerm oil	136
sunflower oil	49
safflower oil	40
sunflower seeds	38

almonds	24
wheatgerm	22
cod liver oil	20
peanut oil	15
tomato purée	5.3
olive oil	5.1
peanut butter	5
egg yolk (raw)	3.1
potato crisps	3.1
spinach	1.7
soya beans	1.1
roasted peanuts	1.1
asparagus	1.1

Cooking tips

Vitamin E is found mainly in vegetable oils, nuts and whole grains such as wheat. Unfortunately, any type of processing of whole grain reduces its vitamin E content. Oatmeal loses only a little as just the hull is removed from the grain, but the refining of white flour leads to 92 per cent of the original vitamin E being lost from the wheat. This is why white bread has so little vitamin E in comparison to brown wholemeal.

Valuable vitamin E supplies are also broken down by oxygen in the air. For example, a bottle of safflower oil stored at room temperature for three months will lose more than half its vitamin E content. This increases if the oil is stored in a warm, light place such as a sunny shelf or window-sill. The best way to preserve the vitamin E content of all foods, including cooking oils, is to store them in a cool, dark larder or fridge.

Cooking, too, results in a significant loss of vitamin E. Commercial cooking at high temperatures, deep-fat frying and deep freezing are the chief culprits. Frying foods can destroy up to 90 per cent of their vitamin E content and frequently happens when the oil or fat in the frying pan is slightly rancid. It is not always easy to tell when a cooking oil has turned rancid, which is why it is best to buy oil in small bottles, store it in a cool, dark place and use it up quickly.

Vitamin E has been shown to block the formation of cancer-causing agents called nitrosamines. These are created by smoked, pickled and cured foods, so if you insist on eating smoky bacon make sure you fry the rashers in a vegetable oil that is rich in vitamin E.

Vitamin E losses		
Food	process	vitamin E loss
tortillas	stored for twelve weeks	95 per cent
wheat	refined to white flour	92 per cent
almonds	roasting	80 per cent
safflower oil	stored for three months	55 per cent
peanut oil	frying for thirty minutes	32 per cent

ACE Vitamins against Smoking

Because the ACE vitamins are all antioxidant nutrients they contain many of the same health properties. It is almost impossible to single out the action of each specific nutrient until much more research into the antioxidants has been completed. For example, the antioxidant nutrients all provide protection for smokers and passive smokers. The damaging effects of smoking are of course well known and we are all aware that smoking is bad news for the body – it causes one third of all deaths in middle age, killing one person in Britain every five minutes.

The metal ions in cigarette smoke destroy our levels of vitamin C. Each cigarette destroys about 25 mg of vitamin C, roughly equivalent to the amount found in a small orange. For this reason smokers risk not having enough vitamin C to remain healthy, and indeed extremely low levels of vitamin C have been found in the bloodstream of smokers, which is probably why they are more likely to develop infections, including coughs, colds and flu. Those who smoke have also been shown to have significantly less beta-carotene in their bloodstream, and as mentioned earlier in this chapter several studies have shown a strong link between low levels of beta-carotene and lung cancer. It seems likely that smokers are running short of beta-carotene even if they do eat up all their greens.

Similarly, smokers are also at risk of low levels of vitamin E. Researchers have found that the fluid in the respiratory tract of smokers contains much less of this vitamin than in non-smokers. Smokers with low levels of this important antioxidant have far less defence against the free radical damage caused by smoking. The obvious answer is to stop smoking and to make sure you live and work in a smoke-free environment. But if this is not possible, all smokers and those forced to breathe in the cigarette smoke of others should seriously consider taking supplements of beta-carotene, vitamin C and vitamin E on a regular basis.

ACE Skin Care

Smokers also have more wrinkles and facial lines than non-smokers. This is probably influenced by insufficient supplies of vitamin C to keep the collagen fibres in the skin in good condition and a lack of vitamin E to repair the free radical damage done to skin cells. Both vitamins C and E not only keep us healthy on the inside but actually keep us young-looking on the outside too. Collagen is an important part of our skin and a good supply of vitamin C boosts collagen supplies which help slow down the formation of facial lines, wrinkles and unattractive skin-slackening. In fact collagen formation is entirely dependent on vitamin C. This is because a substance called hydroxyproline, made in the body by vitamin C and the amino-acid proline, is the major constituent of collagen.

Because of its powers of skin rejuvenation, skin care scientists are trying to use vitamin C in moisturizing creams. However, this vitamin is a highly unstable molecule and cannot easily be added to skin care formulas. Vitamin E-enriched moisturizers are a safer bet when it comes to skin care. Vitamin E may play a vital role in preventing and repairing the free radical damage that creates fine facial lines and wrinkles. Fortunately, vitamin E has a sufficiently small molecular structure to slip through the uppermost layers of skin cells and help repair damaged tissues, which is why it may be helpful in some cases of serious burns, and in wound-healing and repairing scar tissue. Anti-ageing skin care is examined more closely in the following chapter, but generally perhaps the most effective option when it comes to caring for the skin is to keep our internal levels of each of the ACE vitamins topped up from within.

The ACE Minerals

In addition to the ACE vitamins there is a group of minerals that help in the fight against free radicals which should not be overlooked. In fact, the body's first line of defence in fighting the damage caused by the free radicals comes from a group of enzymes that contain the minerals manganese, copper, zinc and selenium. Enzymes control all the chemical changes that take place in our cells, including the creation and release of the energy that keeps the body ticking. Enzymes are catalysts, so they work by speeding up a chemical process, but they need to be triggered into action by several minerals before they can get to work. Outside the body enzymes are often triggered by heat – for example, yeast needs a warm environment before it makes bread rise. However, heat cannot be used inside the body as it would damage the cells. This is where the minerals come in, being used to boost the action of various enzymes. This makes these often overlooked minerals very important elements in our lives.

Manganese

This element is an integral part of life on earth and can even be found in the earth's crust. It is found in tiny quantities in water, plants, animals and humans. The human body contains around 12-20 mg manganese in total, most of this being deposited in the bones, pancreas and liver. However, we lose some of our manganese supply every day through the process of excretion, so to compensate, we need to obtain regular amounts from our diet. Manganese has many functions within the body and helps regulate our growth while maintaining a healthy nervous system, bone development and brain functioning. It is also an essential part of the genetic code contained within all our cells. Manganese is an especially useful weapon in the war against free radicals because it is a component of the enzyme caled superoxide dismutase (known as SOD for short!). This enzyme has the power to react with free radicals and de-activate them, rendering them harmless within the system.

Manganese against disease

Manganese is also important because it is involved with the creation of interferon, an anti-viral and perhaps even anti-cancer compound agent produced by the body in response to disease-producing viruses. Manganese is a vital ingredient, too, in the creation of glycoproteins. These are combinations of glucose and proteins that provide a coating for every cell in the body, protecting them from attacks from free radicals. Some nutritionists have suggested that manganese is especially useful in the fight against arthritis. This is because it is involved in the formation of healthy connective tissue in the joints, and the degeneration of this tissue is a factor in arthritis. A low level of manganese has also been found in patients with heart disease and in diabetics. Some studies into diabetes show that the high blood-sugar levels associated with diabetes may be lowered after treatment with manganese supplements.

How to measure manganese

Manganese is measured in milligrams (mg) and no recommended daily allowance (RDA) has yet been established in Britain. In America, the RDA for adults is between 2 and 5 mg. Those eating a largely vegetarian diet that is rich in whole grains, nuts and seeds are unlikely to run short of manganese.

Where to find manganese			
Food	mg per 100 g	Food	mg per 100 g
wheatgerm	12	almonds	1.7
hazelnuts	4.9	brown rice (boiled)	0.9
wholemeal bread	1.9	beetroot	0.7

Our best sources of manganese are wholegrain cereals and nuts. Manganese is principally found in wheatgerm – this husk is removed from the wheat during refining, which is why white bread contains only one-sixth of the manganese found in wholemeal bread. Manganese is also present in tea and those who drink six or more cups a day are at least supplementing their diet with useful levels. Manganese is one of the safest minerals to add to the diet as any excess the body does not require is simply excreted.

Copper

The name copper comes from the Latin *cuprum*. It is an essential element for life on the planet Earth, for humans, animals and most plants. Copper is all around us, in both the Earth's crust and the sea-water that fills the oceans. Although it is vitally important for our existence, only tiny traces of copper are needed in the human body. For this reason it is known as a trace element.

Copper is stored throughout the body in our blood, bones and liver. It is also a component of many enzymes present in cells, including superoxide dismutase (SOD) which combats free radicals. In addition to its antioxidant properties, copper also protects us from respiratory problems and infections, and is needed for the production of haemoglobin in our red blood cells. Copper is a part of the skin proteins collagen and elastin and is important for maintaining a clear, smooth complexion. It is also needed to make the pigment melanin that colours our skin and hair. Copper is plentiful in many fresh foods, including whole grains, beans, peas and green leafy vegetables and it is rare to suffer from a deficiency of copper, although this can be a cause of anaemia. Many people who suffer from arthritis maintain that wearing a copper bracelet on their wrist reduces pain and inflammation of the joints. There is some medical evidence to support this, as traces of copper do dissolve in the skin's acid secretions and become absorbed into the bloodstream. Such additional copper supplies may help prevent arthritis from taking a hold and in some cases reduce the severity of symptoms.

How to measure copper

Copper is measured in milligrams (mg) and the government guidelines for the intake of copper in adults is 1.2 mg daily. The National Research Council for Food and Nutrition in America recommend a daily intake of between 1.5 and 3 mg. Copper deficiency, while rare, has been seen to occur in those who do not eat enough copper-rich foods such as nuts, wholegrain cereals, wholemeal bread and vegetables such as carrots. Vitamin C is also known to interfere with the absorption of copper, so anyone taking high doses of vitamin C would be wise to balance this with a multi-mineral supplement that contains copper.

Where to find copper

Food	mg per 100 g	Food	mg per 100 g
liver (fried)	12	lentils (boiled)	0.3
crab (boiled)	4.8	olives	0.2
hazelnuts	1.2		

Zinc

Although we only need tiny amounts of zinc it is an essential mineral for maintaining good health. Zinc acts as a traffic controller in the body, directing and overseeing the flow of body processes and the maintenance of all our cells. It is found in tissues throughout the body and is an integral part of the DNA that gives life to our cells. Zinc is essential in other ways as it is needed to make both the male sperm and the female ovum. The developing foetus also requires zinc to ensure healthy bones, brain and nervous system. Zinc is important, too, for converting food into energy and helps in the formation of insulin. It teams up with calcium to strengthen our bones and helps to prevent osteoporosis or softening of the skeleton. Zinc plays a part in the production of over eighty enzymes and hormones in the body, so it is not surprising that a lack of this mineral should have widespread effects. The body is able to store reasonable amounts of zinc, although we do rely on eating regular amounts in our diet. Too much zinc can cause nausea and fever, but too little will stunt growth and harm the immune system. As well as protecting us from within, zinc also makes an important contribution to keeping our skin smooth, supple and blemish-free. Studies by Dr Michaelsson of Upssala University in Sweden into the relationship between zinc and the skin have revealed that in the treatment of a number of skin conditions, notably acne, prescribing zinc supplements can be as beneficial as some antibiotic treatments.

How to measure zinc

Zinc is measured in milligrams (mg) and as yet there is no recommended daily allowance in Britain. However, the European recommendation for zinc in adults is 15 mg. Unfortunately, studies in Britain show that our average daily intake is only around 10.5 mg a day. Zinc is a safe, non-toxic trace mineral – daily doses of 150 mg zinc have been used therapeutically by researchers without ill-effects. However, these large doses should only be taken under professional guidance. Most cases of zinc poisoning occur as a result of inhaling concentrated zinc fumes from an industrial smelting plant. Low levels of zinc have been noted in disorders as diverse as acne, psoriasis, hyperactivity and schizophrenia. Many factors decrease the amount of zinc available for the body to use, including the use of drugs such as the contraceptive pill and steroids, smoking and drinking alcohol. Heavy smokers or drinkers should consider taking a daily zinc supplement, as should diabetics and pregnant and breast-feeding women who are not eating a well-balanced diet high in zinc-rich foods.

Where to find zinc

Food	mg per 100 g	Food	mg per 100 g
calves' liver (fried)	6	tinned ham	2.3
roast beef	5	wholemeal bread	2
chicken liver (fried)	3.4	roast chicken	1.5
sardines	3	boiled eggs	1.3
low-fat Cheddar cheese	2.8	peas	1
Brie	2.7	white bread	0.5
shrimps (tinned)	2.4		

Although zinc can be found in bread and other foods made from wheat, such as pasta, these also contain phytates which bind with minerals such as zinc making them unavailable to the body. For this reason other sources such as meat and vegetables are better foods for keeping our zinc levels high. Vegans may be at risk of a zinc deficiency as they do not eat meat, fish or any dairy products and tend to have a greater intake of foods such as bread, pasta and textured vegetable protein (TVP), all of which have high levels of phytates. In addition to phytates in grains, food refining also strips zinc from our foods. Brown rice contains six times as much zinc as the polished, white varieties. The level of zinc in the soil has also been systematically reduced over the years by intensive farming techniques, which has led to lower levels in crops, including wheat and root vegetables.

Selenium

This little-known mineral is a giant in nutritional terms and has many functions within the body, including a role in protecting us from heart disease and cancer. It is named after the moon goddess Selene who was a charioteer and important in Greek witchcraft (the head of one of her chariot's horses is among the Elgin marbles). Today, the role of selenium in our diet goes beyond witchcraft and is backed by modern science. Large doses of selenium are poisonous and it was only in 1957 that researchers at the University of California discovered the mineral's usefulness in preventing liver damage. Now selenium is recognized by scientists and nutritionists alike as being an essential part of our diet.

We need only tiny quantities of selenium but it has many uses in the body. It keeps the liver functioning healthily, boosts the immune system by protecting our white blood cells, and maintains healthy eyes, skin, hair and heart performance. Selenium is a component of semen and plays an essential role in fertility. It also acts as one of the body's dustmen, removing toxic cadmium and mercury from the body (essential if you are a smoker or breathe in other forms of polluted air). Selenium is a vital component of the enzyme glutathione peroxidase which helps to prevent damage from free radicals. It occurs naturally in some types of soil and is found in whole grains and root vegetables. It is also found in meat, although the levels depend very much on the amount of selenium in the soil on which the animal has been grazing. Blood tests show that in areas with the richest soil the average adult has higher levels of selenium than those who eat a poor diet or live in an area with low selenium levels in the earth. Areas of North America such as Wyoming and the Dakotas have high levels of selenium in their soil, making their grain some of the most nutritious in the world. Other countries, such as Finland and New Zealand, have low levels of selenium and this has been linked to a higher rate of heart disease and cancer. Some parts of Europe are losing selenium from their soils at an alarming rate. In Sweden, the government is so concerned about the problem that they now offer a free daily supplement to all pregnant women. There is now concern that British soil is also falling below a safe nutritional standard: Norfolk, for example, used to have some of the highest supplies of selenium in its soil, but these have been falling steadily since the advent of intensive farming methods and the over-use of fertilizers. Studies show that on average our daily intake has dropped from 60 mcg a day in 1975 to 35 mcg and below today. This may be because since joining the EC, we now import a softer European wheat that is low in selenium, instead of the hard American grain that has higher levels.

Selenium and other nutrients

An unusual feature of selenium is that it boosts the powers of other vitamins within the system. When selenium is linked with vitamin E in the body, the vitamin lasts longer and is able to work harder. Selenium and vitamin E work synergistically, that is to say, they have a greater effect working together than they do separately. Protective enzymes produced in the body also need both selenium and vitamin E to function effectively. In addition, studies on cancer in animals show that selenium increases the potency of vitamins C and E, and that it may give better relief from angina (chest pains) than using vitamin E on its own.

How to measure selenium

Selenium is a trace mineral and small quantities are needed by the body for overall good health. For this reason it is measured in micrograms (mcg). As yet, there is no RDA of selenium in Britain. However, it is thought that we need 1-2 mcg for each kilo of body weight. The average adult weighing 70 kilos therefore requires a daily intake of 70-140 mcg. The safe and adequate intake recommended by the World Health Organization is 50-200 mcg a day. A substantial excess of selenium can cause birth defects, hair loss and blotchy skin. Selenium poisoning is unlikely to occur from our food but is possible if far too many supplements are taken. Government figures suggest that the maximum daily intake of selenium from all sources, including food, should not exceed 450 mcg.

Where to find selenium

Food	mcg per 100 g	Food	mcg per 100 g
wholemeal flour	53	boiled eggs	11
shrimps (tinned)	52	mushrooms (raw)	9
shrimps (frozen)	49	wheatbran	9
strong white flour	42	white rice (boiled)	4
green/brown lentils (boiled)	40	macaroni (boiled)	4
crab (boiled)	17	beef steak	3
low-fat Cheddar cheese	15		

The level of selenium in foods varies considerably depending on selenium levels in the soil. Cattle grazed on poor soil will not absorb much of the mineral from the grass and so will not contain much in their milk or meat. Likewise, eggs from chickens that have not been allowed to feed on selenium-rich foods will not contain as much as the well-fed free-range birds. So buying free-range eggs is not only better for the birds, but can be of benefit to our bodies too. Brewer's yeast is also a good source of selenium and is especially useful for vegetarians and vegans.

Selenium exists in several forms; organic selenium, best absorbed by the body, is included in some mineral supplements and is made by growing yeast in a selenium-enriched medium. This ensures that the yeast absorbs the organic selenium into its cells. Inorganic selenium, such as sodium selenite, seems to be less easily absorbed by the body and is more toxic if taken in excess.

The ACE Team

There is now no doubt in the minds of the world's scientists and doctors that the ACE vitamins are essential to maintain good health. Studies indicate that, overall, vitamin E is probably the most important antioxidant as it protects the fats that surround every single living cell. Vitamin E may also play the most significant role in the fight against heart disease, Britain's number one killer. However, beta-carotene is likely to be especially useful in combating cancer, and vitamin C is extremely helpful in maintaining our immune system, and backs up the action of vitamin E. In short, the ACE vitamins all work together to keep us fit and healthy. As the months go by and further trials are concluded, there is increasing evidence that the ACE vitamins prevent serious diseases and put ageing on hold.

3

ACTIVE ANTI-AGEING

The idea that the ACE vitamins can slow down the ageing process is exciting scientists all over the world. Preliminary research suggests that by increasing our intake of beta-carotene, vitamins C and E, we can help ward off many of the diseases associated with growing old. While the ACE vitamins are unlikely to turn back the hands on the clock, they do seem able to slow down its ticking. There is nothing wrong with growing older as such, of course, indeed from the very moment we are born the ageing process begins, but there are obvious drawbacks when the process of ageing affects our health and well-being. Most of us probably don't think much about growing older until our bodies begin to change. Our system starts to slow down, we become less energetic, our vision blurs, our skin becomes wrinkled and our hair turns grey. Exactly what causes these changes is not yet clear, but scientists now know that free radical activity plays an integral part in the ageing process, and can be counteracted by the ACE vitamins.

Basically, there are two types of ageing. The first is the natural, chronological state of growing older which happens to us all. There is not a lot that we can do to influence this and, if we are lucky with our genes, we can remain fit and active until the end of our lives. The second type is premature, degenerative ageing. This is when we develop the diseases such as arthritis and cataracts that so often plague the elderly. Nutritional science now offers us a chance to slow down premature ageing and improve the quality of life in old age. Our main adversaries in the ageing process are believed to be the free radicals that occur as a result of oxidation. By helping to control these, we may be able to delay the onset of many diseases associated with ageing, including heart disease, cancer, Parkinson's disease and lowered immunity, and may even remain looking youthful by warding off the wrinkles.

Radical Tactics

Growing evidence suggests that it is an imbalance of free radicals that makes us age and die before our time. Scientific studies are also indicating that the antioxidant ACE vitamins can slow down, and in some cases may even reverse, the degenerative ageing process. The implications of this news are enormous as the number of elderly people in Britain is rapidly growing. By the end of this decade more than a million Britons will be over the age of eighty-five. This trend looks set to continue and we will be increasingly faced with the problems of an ageing population. Typical disorders include poor eyesight and blindness due to cataracts; swollen, painful joints and immobility due to arthritis, and breathing difficulties such as emphysema. These have all been linked to the destructive nature of free radicals. 'Free radical damage is a very important part of the ageing process – much more important than scientists were willing to accept in the past', says Dr Earl Stadtman, head of biochemistry at the National Heart, Lung and Blood Institute in the USA.

One of the first scientists to link free radical damage with ageing was Professor Denham Harman, based at the University of Nebraska. He voiced the idea as long ago as 1954, insisting:

'Ageing is the ever-increasing accumulation of changes

caused or contributed to by free radicals.'

Laboratory research confirms that when cells die, almost a third of their proteins are damaged beyond repair by free radical attack. According to the respected cancer researcher Dr Bruce Ames at the University of California, each human cell receives at least 10,000 damaging 'hits' from free radicals every day. Normally the body can repair the damage by using its own supply of enzymes and other proteins. But as we get older, this inbuilt ability to repair our cells is reduced. Fortunately, nature gives us an antidote in the form of the antioxidant ACE vitamins. By eating more of these vitamins in everyday foods such as fruits, vegetables and whole grains, we may be better equipped to enjoy our retirement.

Clinical trials are currently underway in many research centres around the world to prove that antioxidants do indeed extend human life. The interim reports are encouraging, but the final results will obviously not be available for many decades. Meanwhile, research by scientists such as Dr Bruce Ames shows that the lifespan of an animal is directly related to its ability to repair free radical damage. Studies at the Scottish Agricultural College show that certain foods have the potential to delay the signs of ageing. Mice fed antioxidant extracts from plants and herbs have been found to live longer. Scientists examining the tissues of these mice found that those who had been fed regular amounts of antioxidants had healthier cells than those who had not received the nutrients. Dr Stanley Deans, who is in charge of this research, says:

'The beneficial effects of the antioxidants are profound because they have anti-ageing properties in animals. We may find in the future they help to reduce all kinds of ageing disorders, such as Alzheimer's disease and skin wrinkling.'

Human trials involving antioxidants in herbal extracts are due to start in 1994. Until these results are known, Dr Deans suggests sprinkling a spoonful of mixed fresh herbs on to every meal to help slow down the ageing process.

Lifespan vs. Life Expectancy

All species have their own lifespan, which is defined as being the maximum length of time they can live. This ranges from three years for mice, to forty-five years for monkeys and around 120 years for human beings. Life expectancy for a species is calculated by the length of time 50 per cent of the population survives. The difference between maximum lifespan and life expectancy depends on environmental and genetic factors. In industrialized countries life expectancy had risen to sixty-seven by 1946, and today it stands at around seventy-four. These increases are largely due to improved hygiene conditions preventing bacterial infections. Very few individuals in the Western world reach their maximum potential of around 120 years. The vast majority die prematurely from diseases involving free radicals.

Free radical damage is a key to the ageing process for many species. Research on such varied creatures as lobsters and fruit-flies has revealed that low levels of free radical activity dramatically increase life expectancy. In the case of the lobster and some of its marine companions such as sea anemones, degenerative ageing appears not to be inevitable. It seems that these sea creatures are protected from free radical damage in some way, and manage to grow old without deteriorating. Earthly creatures such as roundworms are also protected from free radical attack by high levels of antioxidants in their system. Researchers at the University of Colorado have bred a strain of roundworm which enjoys a 65% increase in lifespan. These long-lived worms have higher than normal amounts of the antioxidants superoxide dismutase (SOD) and catalase. 'That's very exciting to a lot of people in the ageing field,' says team leader Professor Thomas Johnson.

The idea of breeding species to extend their lifespan looks like becoming a reality in the not too distant future. According to Professor Michael Rose at the University of California, there is, for the first time, 'a real possibility of affecting the ageing process with bio-medical intervention.' Speaking at the American Association for the

Advancement of Science in 1992, Professor Rose said: 'There is nothing deeply problematic about doubling the human lifespan. Ageing used to be mysterious and now it isn't. It is a problem that has been solved.' Scientists at the University of California have bred fruit-flies that can live the equivalent of about 150 human years. The genes of these flies contain the antioxidant SOD that neutralizes free radicals and prevents cell damage.

Free radicals are also involved in other research into slowing down the ageing process. It has been known for several years that rats fed a restricted diet live longer than those allowed to eat what they choose. One reason for this may be that the rats on a low-calorie diet keep their proteins turning over at a higher rate than normal. This could help them cope better with the ageing effects of protein damage caused by free radicals. Whichever theory is proved to be right, it seems that the action of free radicals will be involved somewhere along the line. This realization has led to a great deal of research into the causes of free radical damage and the tremendous anti-ageing potential of the ACE vitamins. Ultimately, says Dr Bruce Ames, 'We're going to be able to get people to live a lot longer than anyone thinks.'

Anti-ageing Vitamins

The Americans are highly expert when it comes to researching the ageing process. The Human Nutrition Research Center on Ageing is housed in an impressive skyscraper in the centre of Boston. Here, elderly volunteers check in for residential nutrition programmes where every mouthful of food is monitored. Those taking part have their blood plasma and urine analysed, and undergo regular fitness checks. The centre is well equipped with comfortable bedrooms, a restaurant, a gym with fine views over Boston harbour and even a swimming-pool on the top floor. Despite the strict restrictions on food and drink, which is carefully controlled down to the nearest gram, there is still a waiting list to participate.

The residential programmes at the Human Nutrition Research Center on Ageing have shed a good deal of light on how the ACE vitamins help delay the ageing process. According to Professor Jeffrey Blumberg, Associate Director, one of the most useful findings is how the antioxidant vitamins boost our immune systems. 'Our immune system responses slow down with age,' he explains, 'but we have found that vitamin E is very important in maintaining an optimum immune response. High doses of vitamin E can stimulate the immune system and may even regenerate it.'

The most recent trials have shown that vitamin E specifically increases the power of the helper T-cells (an essential type of white blood cell) and also boosts the production of antibodies. As we age, so our ability to ward off infection is gradually diminished. We produce fewer of the infection-fighting white blood cells which is why the elderly are most susceptible to invading bacteria, viruses and other germs. This also explains why life-threatening diseases such as cancer are more common among the elderly. Some researchers are suggesting that the low levels of white blood cells seen in the elderly are due to the life-long process of oxidation and production of free radicals. Studies at the Human Nutrition Research Center on Ageing involved giving elderly volunteers a large daily dose of vitamin E capsules (totalling 800 IU). When blood samples were analysed for several measures of immune response, those volunteers who had regularly taken the vitamin were seen to have an improved immune function compared to those who had been given dummy supplements. In this case, cells were better able to communicate among themselves, which meant that they could be more effective in fighting disease. Beta-carotene has also been shown to boost the immune system and even reduce the size of cancerous tumours in animals. There is strong evidence that beta-carotene enhances many aspects of immunity and that a diet rich in carotenoids is linked to a lower risk of developing many types of cancer.

Studies published in *The Lancet* in 1992 also show that

the ACE vitamins boost the immune system. Research conducted by Professor Ranjit Chandra at the World Health Organization for Nutritional Immunology tested the ACE vitamins on ninety-six healthy elderly volunteers. Two groups of individuals were involved in the trial. The first were given a daily dose of vitamins A, C, D and E, B-complex vitamins, beta-carotene, folic acid, iron, zinc, copper, selenium, iodine, calcium and magnesium. The quantities given were similar to the recommended daily allowances, except for vitamin E and beta-carotene which were much greater. The second set of patients were given a dummy supplement containing only calcium and magnesium. Both groups took the supplements every day for twelve months. At the end of the trial, those who had taken the supplements that included the ACE vitamins saw a 'significant improvement in several immune responses'. Professor Chandra concludes that the results of this study substantiate the theory that our nutritional status directly relates to our well-being, and that by taking vitamin supplements we can increase our immunity: 'Such an intervention led to a striking reduction in illness – a find that is of considerable clinical and public health importance.'

The evidence suggests that taking vitamin supplements does no harm and has enormous potential in controlling many crippling and costly chronic diseases. Professor Blumberg at the Human Nutrition Research Center on Ageing sums up by saying, 'I think we have enough data in hand for physicians to begin suggesting their patients take supplements, or at least not discourage them from it.' As he so aptly points out: 'No one seems to mind prescribing endless drugs for the elderly, so why not an inexpensive and safe nutrient?'

Cataracts

The condition of cataracts is the world's number one cause of blindness and mainly affects the elderly. As many as half the population who are aged seventy-five or over will suffer from this disorder, which causes a clouding of the eye lens and results in poor vision or even blindness in later life. The good news is that those in middle age who eat plenty of carrots, spinach and orange juice can dramatically reduce their risk of cataracts. Beta-carotene together with vitamins C and E appears to slow down chemical changes in the eye lens.

When light is absorbed by the eye, it generates oxyradicals, a particularly active form of free radical. Oxyradicals appear to promote the formation of opacities on the lens, a type of protein that clouds the vision. The gelatine-like cells of the eyes, which are normally clear, become damaged, and tiny droplets of fat leak out. Oxyradicals also suppress the function of the enzymes that would normally get rid of these damaged proteins. Like dirt on a camera lens, these tiny particles block the vision and make the eyes look cloudy. The oxidation of cells in the lens by free radicals, the main cause of cataracts, is thought to be the result of ultra-violet rays from sunlight. Researchers have been looking at the role of the ACE vitamins in preventing this disorder.

Supplements of vitamin E have been shown to slow down the rate of cataracts forming, or even prevent them altogether. One study at the University of Western Ontario in Canada found that those who took vitamin E supplements averaging 400 IU a day were half as likely to develop cataracts as those who did not. Those who took a mixture of both vitamins C and E cut their risk by two-thirds. Dr James Robertson, who conducted the Canadian trial, says that 'this information could have a large impact on the incidence of cataracts in older people'. As a follow-up study, he is now investigating an 'antioxidant cocktail' containing each of the ACE vitamins as a way of protecting the eyes against the formation of cataracts. Interestingly, studies that dose patients with vitamin C lead to high levels of this vitamin being found in the eye lens, which indicates that the body sends it there to give some kind of protection.

Thus American research suggests that vitamin supplements may reduce the numbers of cataracts caused by ageing by at least half, and while other scientists have concluded that vitamins C and E may not actually prevent cataracts from occurring, they do agree that they seem to delay their onset and development.

The Brain Drain

One of the most distressing problems of old age is Alzheimer's disease. This tragic affliction causes the elderly to lose their memory, and become confused, dazed and disoriented. Alzheimer's disease can become a living nightmare for the many carers who look after elderly relatives. Sufferers have to be looked after every minute of the day and there is currently no way to improve their situation. There is no known cure for Alzheimer's disease and scientists are still a long way from pin-pointing its cause. However, French researchers have shown that some Alzheimer's sufferers have low levels of the ACE vitamins in their bloodstream, which could be a contributory factor. High levels of aluminium in the bloodstream is another popular theory as aluminosilicate deposits are found in the brains of Alzheimer's victims, and scientists at the Dunn Nutrition Centre in Cambridge are investigating whether these deposits might involve free radicals. The brain cells of mice have shown that free radicals and oxygen-derived metabolites are produced during the build-up of aluminium levels in the brain.

The activity of free radicals within the brain is another notion that is gaining ground. Free radicals damage brain cells much as they do other cells in the body. They attack the fats that surround brain cells and disrupt delicate tissues. Autopsies on elderly people show that their brain cells are more damaged by oxidation from free radicals than those in young people. It is difficult to carry out experiments on living human brain cells, so scientists turn instead to laboratory rodents for their research. Scientists at the Oklahoma Medical Research Foundation have discovered that free radicals reduce the short-term memory of gerbils. This can be tested by putting gerbils in a small maze and recording how many mistakes they make as they attempt to find their way out. When elderly gerbils were placed in the maze they initially took twice as many wrong turnings as the younger gerbils, who had memorized their escape route. But after doses of antioxidants, the elderly group of gerbils were able to leave the maze as quickly as the younger group. When the antioxidant treatment was stopped, their earlier forgetfulness returned. This simple piece of research gives us hope that humans may also be able to overcome memory loss with the help of the ACE vitamins.

Parkinson's Disease
Parkinson's disease is another crippling brain disorder that can strike at any age, but most often affects the middle-aged and elderly. Parkinson's disease stems from a malfunction in the brain cells that control movement. These cells produce a chemical called dopamine that is essential for the brain to send messages to muscles. As the brain cells die and dopamine levels drop, patients are left with trembling hands and limbs, a shuffling walk and an inability to control their actions. Although we do not know what causes these brain cells to die, some researchers believe that it may be due to oxidation and the action of free radicals. To test this theory, scientists have turned to the antioxidant ACE vitamins.

Several studies have linked low levels of vitamin C with Parkinson's disease. One study, conducted by the Bury Health Authority in Lancashire, assessed 100 elderly people entering residential homes. They were screened for signs of early Parkinson's disease and for vitamin C deficiency. The prevalence of Parkinson's disease was much higher in those with low levels of vitamin C. More research needs to be done, but there is increasing evidence to suggest that the antioxidant action of vitamin C protects nerve cells against damage.

The main drug used to treat Parkinson's disease is levodopa, which loses its effectiveness with prolonged use. For this reason, it is often best to delay drug treatment for as long as possible. With this in mind, a study of the factors that cause the nerve cell degeneration seen in Parkinson's disease was carried out at the Neurological Institute of New York. Patients with early signs of Parkinson's disease were advised to take high-dose supplements of vitamin E (3200 IU a day) and vitamin C (3000 mg a day). The patients were not yet taking levodopa, although they were taking other drugs in an attempt to delay levodopa therapy. A similar group of patients was managed in the same way, except that they did not receive the antioxidant vitamins. The time when levodopa became necessary was extended by two and a half years in the patients who were receiving the vitamins, as compared to those who were not. However, a recent follow-up study showed that vitamin E was not effective, so the results are not conclusive.

Foods rich in the ACE vitamins may also be helpful in slowing down the symptoms of Parkinson's disease. Studies at the University of Medicine at New Jersey compared eighty-one Parkinson's patients with a brother or sister of the same sex without the disease, and it was found that those who ate the most walnuts, sunflower seeds, vegetable oil and plums had the least incidence of Parkinson's disease. Nuts, seeds and oils are all excellent sources of vitamin E. Plums contain only reasonable amounts, but are one of the best fruit sources of this vitamin. Further studies are now underway to establish the precise role of the ACE vitamins in the fight against Parkinson's disease.

Exercise

Muscles throughout the body can become damaged beyond repair in old age as a result of the ill-effects of free radicals and the subsequent oxidation of cells. One of the first signs of growing older is loss of energy, suppleness and strength. Active sports such as tennis, squash and athletics give way to less physically demanding pursuits such as golf and bowls. However, encouraging preliminary research suggests that vitamin E reduces the muscle deterioration that usually accompanies old age.

Researchers in Boston looked at twenty-one fit young and older men who took part in an extensive exercise programme. At the same time, the men were given either a large dose of vitamin E (800 IU) or a dummy supplement each day. To measure the amount of muscle damage, the researchers looked at the by-products of fat oxidation in urine samples and took small tissue biopsies from leg muscles. Those who had been given the daily dose of vitamin E showed less exercise-induced muscle damage when compared to the others. They had fewer signs of cell damage due to oxidation and reduced levels of two chemical messengers that cause inflammation in the tissues. 'The older men seem to benefit the most,' noted Professor Mohsen Meydani, who was in charge of the trial. One way the vitamin is thought to take effect is by preventing the damage to muscle-cell membranes caused by oxygen while working out. As vitamin E is also known to help prevent muscle damage and post-exercise stiffness, it may be helpful to increase our intake to maintain optimum activity in old age.

Arthritis

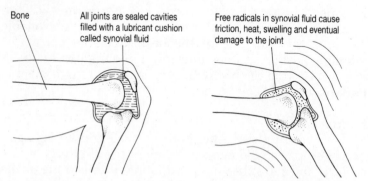

Bone

All joints are sealed cavities filled with a lubricant cushion called synovial fluid

Free radicals in synovial fluid cause friction, heat, swelling and eventual damage to the joint

Many elderly people find their mobility becomes increasingly restricted with age. There are two basic forms of arthritis: the most frequent is osteoarthritis and the less common is rheumatoid arthritis. Osteoarthritis is a 'wear and tear' disorder of the joint cartilage, associated with changes in the underlying bone which cause joint problems. The parts of the body most frequently affected are the hip, knee and thumb joints. Osteoarthritis may also be caused by overuse of a certain joint, such as the knees and feet of athletes. This form of arthritis can be picked up by X-rays which reveal the narrowing of the joint spaces due to cartilage loss. Rheumatoid arthritis is linked to damage to the immune system and is detected by a blood test, which shows the presence of the rheumatoid factor, and also by X-rays which reveal changes around the affected joints. Less is known about rheumatoid arthritis, but it is thought to be linked to genetic disorders, diet and certain types of infection.

The term 'arthritic' is used to describe any kind of sore, stiff or aching joints. There may be several reasons why this soreness occurs, but the underlying cause in all cases is inflammation within the joints. The symptoms in each case are similar, too: pain, swelling, warmth, redness of the overlying skin, joint deformities and restricted mobility. One of the most important clues in seeking a cure for arthritis is the action of free radicals within the body. Internal inflammation is almost always triggered by free radical activity, so the theory is that antioxidant nutrients may be able to reduce or even prevent this. Within the joints there is a lubricant called synovial fluid which 'oils' the joints and allows them to move freely. When free radicals get into the synovial fluid they cause it to lose its lubricating properties by oxidizing the fats in the fluid. Once it has been damaged in this way the synovial fluid is unable to lubricate the joints effectively and the result is severe inflammation. In a report published in the *American Journal of Clinical Nutrition* in 1992, researchers at the London Hospital found that 'lipid peroxidation of the cell membranes results in a decrease in membrane fluidity . . . these pathological changes result in tissue inflammation. Thus there is a sound rationale for antioxidant therapy.'

The ACE vitamins may have an important role in neutralizing the excess levels of free radicals that damage the synovial fluid in the joints. Many people with arthritis report that their symptoms subside if they switch to a wholefood diet that is rich in fresh fruits and vegetables and low in processed refined foods. One reason for this may be that by doing so, they are automatically boosting their levels of the ACE vitamins, and certainly many nutritionists believe that diet plays a key role in the long-term control of this debilitating disease.

A study reported in *The Lancet* in 1991 describes how arthritic patients on a one-year vegetarian diet benefited from reduced swelling, greater mobility of the joints and a stronger grip. The special diet started with a week-long fast during which patients took only herbal teas, garlic, vegetable broth and juice extracts from carrots, beets and celery. After their fast, patients were put on an 'exclusion' diet where foods were introduced one at a time to identify any allergic reactions. Wheat, citrus fruits, sugar and dairy products are all believed to provoke the symptoms of arthritis. To boost their frugal diet, the volunteers were given food supplements, including a daily dose of beta-carotene, vitamin C and vitamin E. At the end of the year, those who had made changes in their diet had greatly improved, while the control group who made no changes got even worse. This study shows that those who boost their intake of the ACE vitamins can improve their condition. Not only did the patients take supplements of beta-carotene and vitamin E, they also increased their intake by drinking carrot juice (rich in beta-carotene) and eating many more fresh fruits and vegetables (rich in vitamin C). Their increased levels of antioxidants are thought to have improved arthritis by keeping down the levels of free radicals in the synovial fluid and maintaining optimum movement. Preventing the build-up of free radicals helps to reduce the symptoms of heat, pain and swelling that they cause.

Studies investigating the role of the ACE vitamins in arthritis reveal that sufferers have low levels of vitamin C. This is possibly because vitamin C is used to fight the free radicals produced within the synovial fluid. Vitamin C is important for keeping mobile as it is a vital part of the cartilage and collagen found in the joints, and some limited research also suggests that vitamin C can help reduce back pain by maintaining the tissues surrounding the discs in the spine. Vitamin E has also been shown to help cases of arthritis. In animals, a lack of vitamin E causes a form of the condition which can be remedied by giving the animals vitamin E supplements, another indicator that it is important to eat sufficient amounts of the ACE vitamins to protect our joints against arthritis. Further studies involving the power of the ACE vitamins to combat serious disorders that most often affect the elderly, including heart disease and cancer, are reviewed in the following chapter.

War on Wrinkles

While the medical world concentrates on life-threatening diseases, the cosmetic industry has been investigating the ACE vitamins for a more aesthetic purpose. An anti-ageing face cream that can wipe away wrinkles is the modern-day equivalent of the elusive Holy Grail. Any moisturizer that guarantees to turn back the clock is also a guaranteed money-spinner. As a result, skin-care scientists have been looking with interest at the use of antioxidant vitamins for several years. The theory is that if the ACE vitamins help repair cells within the body, they should also be able to restore damaged skin cells on its surface. As a result, some of the jargon that was previously confined to biochemisty laboratories has been creeping on to the cosmetic counters. Pick up any jar of highly priced and expensively packaged moisturizer and the chances are that it will mention the scourge of free radicals and the skin-saving properties of vitamin E. But do the creams that contain antioxidants really make any difference to facial lines?

One of the world's leading skin scientists is convinced that they do. Dr Daniel Maes is a director of research and development for Estee Lauder in New York. He has made skin-care science his specialized subject and is recognized as being one of the best in the business. Although employed by a commercial company, he regularly shares his research with medical organizations around the globe. Dr Maes believes that all premature lines and wrinkles are caused by free radicals. 'There is no doubt that the action of free radicals is what causes our skin to wrinkle and sag over time,' he states. 'The key for us as a cosmetic company is to find an answer to the destructive properties of free radicals within the skin.'

Radical skin damage

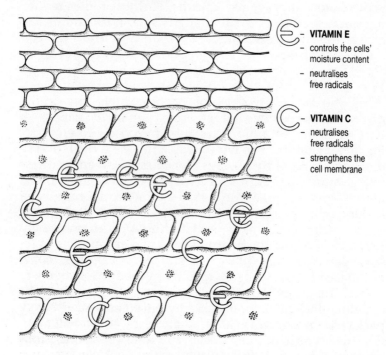

VITAMIN E
- controls the cells' moisture content
- neutralises free radicals

VITAMIN C
- neutralises free radicals
- strengthens the cell membrane

The skin's main function is to protect the body within and in doing so it comes under constant attack from free radicals. The main sources of free radical attack on the skin are sunlight and pollution. Every time we step outdoors our skin is subjected to increased levels of ageing free radicals from the ultra-violet sun's rays. These UV rays are stronger when the sun is shining or if we expose our skin to the sun without first applying a protective sunblock cream. Free radicals are also created within the skin as a result of pollutants (including car fumes and cigarette smoke) that settle on the skin's surface.

Free radicals actively damage the skin in several different ways. They destroy the membranes surrounding the skin cells, causing the contents to leak out and disintegrate. They also encourage the breakdown of the collagen and elastin fibres that support the skin. Without this underlying support, the complexion begins to slacken and sag. The first signs of skin ageing can be seen as early as the mid-twenties. This is when crow's feet start to form around the eyes and tiny wrinkles appear on the forehead. From then on the complexion slides, quite literally, downhill. The effects of gravity tend to pull the skin downwards and the action of free radicals within the skin encourages a visible loss of elasticity and tone. The antioxidant nutrients such as vitamin E and beta-carotene help mop up most of the free radicals linked to such destruction, while vitamin C is useful for stimulating the fibroblast cells to produce more collagen which supports the skin and keeps the complexion smooth.

Other skin problems also increase with age. UV radiation from the sun encourages freckling, uneven pigmentation and lipofuscin, known as 'liver spots' or 'age spots', which often appear on the face and the backs of the hands, sometimes as early as the age of thirty. These age spots, which once with you will not disappear, are thought to be the end-products of free radical reactions in the body and can be prevented by the daily use of a sunblock. Increased levels of vitamin E have also been shown to help. In a study of 200 elderly people, half were given a daily dose of vitamin E and other antioxidants, while the remainder were supplied with dummy supplements. After one year, those who had been given the vitamins had fewer patches of increased pigmentation and less noticeable age spots.

Vitamin E also protects the skin against other damage from the sun. Laboratory tests on synthetic skin show that when it is subjected to UV light cells are destroyed. However, if the synthetic skin is first coated with a layer of vitamin E, the signs of free radical inflammation are greatly reduced. Further studies show vitamin E to be a potent wrinkle-reducer and skin conditioner. In trials carried out over a four-week period, twenty women aged between forty-two and sixty-four years tested the effectiveness of a cream containing 5 per cent natural vitamin E. The cream was applied daily to the corner of one eyelid, while the corner of the other eye was treated with a similar cream that did not contain any vitamin E. At the end of the month, an imprint of the skin was taken and a three-dimensional image made to show the depth of wrinkles surrounding each eyelid. More than half the women treated saw a visible improvement in the depth of their crow's feet after using the vitamin E cream. There was no discernible difference in the skin that had the applications of plain cream. Researchers noted that the active cream encouraged a significant decrease in the length and depth of the wrinkles. The study concluded: 'When used in skin-care products, natural vitamin E will protect the skin from ultra-violet light, reduce the appearance of fine facial lines and wrinkles, and help delay the progression of ageing.'

Wrinkle-reducers

Each of the ACE vitamins has great potential for keeping the complexion youthful as they protect the cells in many different ways. In addition to outside influences such as sunshine and pollution, our skin is also damaged by elements from within the body. As our skin ages, it becomes more susceptible to attack from certain enzymes such as collagenase. This enzyme is encouraged by free radicals and can cut up and destroy collagen fibres, leading to wrinkles. Another enzyme that can damage the skin is elastase. This may destroy the elastin fibres in the skin and also lead to skin sagging and wrinkles. Both collagenase and elastase occur naturally and a certain amount is essential for strong, supple skin. However, their activity is increased by ultra-violet light and cigarette smoke, including passive smoking. As we get older, we are more at risk, as it takes less sunlight to activate the high levels of enzymes that may damage the skin. Fortunately, vitamin C is involved with these enzymes and may help regulate their action within the skin.

From a purely cosmetic point of view, we should increase our intake of vitamin C as we get older. As mentioned in the previous chapter, skin-care scientists are also looking at ways of including vitamin C in skin creams, but this is difficult as vitamin C is easily oxidized and readily inactivated. It is impossible to stir vitamin C into a skin cream as it would react with the other ingredients and break down. Cosmetic scientists have found a way of coating molecules of vitamin C before adding them to a moisturizer, but this is time-consuming and expensive. A few sophisticated formulations manage to combine vitamin C and vitamin E, a duo which is more effective in controlling the formation of wrinkles than vitamin C alone. Beta-carotene is also being studied for inclusion in skin-care products, but the main problem is that it stains the skin yellow. Experiments are now underway with a bleached version of beta-carotene, but it is not yet clear how effective this will be. For the time being, moisturizing creams that contain vitamins C and E are the most promising for actually reducing the formation of fine lines and wrinkles. Taking regular doses of the ACE vitamins is another way of protecting the skin, but the doses do need to be relatively high. This is because the transfer rate of vitamins from the liver to the skin is poor, as the nutrients are used up in other more important functions en route. Using a vitamin-enriched moisturizing skin cream delivers the antioxidants directly to the skin's surface where they form a protective buffer-zone against environmental damage. Look for the words 'alpha tocopherol', which means vitamin E, amongst the ingredients or squeeze the contents of a vitamin E capsule into a jar of your favourite brand of moisturizer.

Ageing on hold

While ageing is inevitable, the frailty, sickness and skin wrinkling that so often accompany it are not. No matter what our age, we can all adopt the ACE Plan ten-point strategy for active anti-ageing.

1. Cut down exposure to pollutants such as cigarette smoke and car exhaust fumes.
2. Eat plenty of vegetables that contain beta-carotene. The best are carrots, spinach and broccoli.
3. Each more fresh fruits rich in vitamin C, such as oranges, grapefruit and strawberries.
4. Eat a wider range of wholegrain foods such as wheat-germ and wholemeal bread that contain vitamin E.
5. Use a cooking oil rich in vitamin E, such as olive oil, for frying foods and making salad dressings.
6. Take a moderate amount of exercise every day – even a short walk around the block is better than nothing.
7. Always apply a sunblock to the face, neck and back of the hands before going outdoors (even when the sun isn't shining).
8. Wear a wide-brimmed hat and long sleeves when in strong sunshine and take extra care not to get sunburnt.
9. Give your body plenty of rest, with at least seven hours' regular sleep each night.
10. Take a daily multi-vitamin supplement of beta-carotene, vitamin C and vitamin E. Alternatively, look for one of the newer antioxidant formulas, especially those containing natural vitamins.

4
MEDICAL MATTERS

Evidence is emerging from laboratories and clinics around the world to suggest that we should reconsider the role of vitamins. 'There are certainly indications that vitamins do more than just prevent deficiency diseases,' says Dr Walter Mertz, director of the USA's Human Nutrition Research Center. Month after month, serious scientific and medical journals are publishing the results of clinical trials on vitamins that have been carried out around the world. Slowly but surely, even the most hardened sceptics are being led to the conclusion that several vitamins play an important role in disease prevention. For example, the Chief Medical Officer now advises that all women of childbearing age (who might become pregnant) should take a daily supplement of folic acid (one of the B vitamins) to help prevent birth defects such as spina bifida. The supplements are recommended because we do not get enough folic acid in our diet to pass on the proven clinical benefit. The ACE vitamins are also believed to help prevent many diseases. Although research is just beginning in this field, the results are already impressive.

Types of study:

There are several different kinds of study that are carried out in the course of research. Some are more noteworthy than others. For example, results observed in a test-tube may not necessarily guarantee the same response in a human being. In order to put the results of medical and scientific studies into perspective, it's useful to understand how the evidence is gathered.

- **Anecdotal evidence:** This is based on personal observations in a laboratory or during clinical procedures.

Pros: Most research starts out as anecdotal evidence which is then expanded and proved by more sophisticated methods.

Cons: Not reliable as the results may be a one-off or involve too few subjects to be statistically significant.

- **In vitro:** This involves testing cells from a living organism in a test-tube or, more commonly, a petri-dish.

Pros: Simple and inexpensive. Gives a good indication of how a substance behaves.

Cons: May not give the same results in a test-tube as would be seen in a human being.

- **In vivo:** This testing is carried out on tissue culture, animals or human volunteers.

Pros: Tests the entire living system and so is a good method of analysis. Today, tissue cultures using living tissues are largely replacing animal experiments. Human tests are even more precise.

Cons: Animal experiments are often cruel and what works for a rat may not automatically help a human. In vivo testing tends to be expensive and takes time. Results are slow, especially in humans, as we have a long life span.

- **Epidemiological studies:** These look at the spread of disease in large populations. Researchers gather vast amounts of information from tens of thousands of people to pick up patterns of disease in relation to diet, lifestyle or other factors.

Pros: Inexpensive. Useful to pick up widespread trends in public health.

Cons: Difficult to pin-point exactly what is responsible for causing the problems that are identified.

- **Clinical trial:** Involves two groups of volunteers, one half is given the active substance and the other half is not given anything. Both groups are monitored and compared at the end of the trial.

Pros: Gives a good indication of whether a substance produces a measurable effect in humans.

Cons: Those who choose to take the tablets may be more aware of their health generally, which could influence the results.

- **Double-blind clinical trial:** In this case, one half of the test group receives the substance being tested, the other half is given a dummy pill (placebo). Neither the researchers nor the volunteers know which they are being given.

Pros: Very reliable results that are entirely objective and not influenced by any subconscious bias. No one who is involved with the trial knows who is taking what, thereby eliminating the chance of any psychological benefit of taking a pill, known as the placebo effect.

Cons: Expensive, time-consuming, and large groups need to be monitored over a long period of time for the research to be statistically significant.

Coronary Heart Disease

Heart disease is the major killer in the modern industrialized world. Almost half the population of Europe will die from heart or circulatory diseases. In Britain, heart disease causes over 160,000 premature deaths every year, which is well over 3000 each week, and a recent government health survey found that nine out of ten Britons run a risk of heart disease or strokes. Although it is mainly thought of as a male disease, it is also the leading cause of death for women. Over 78,000 women die every year from heart disease, a statistic which contrasts dramatically with deaths from breast cancer (15,000), ovarian cancer (4000) and cervical cancer (2000). Few of us can afford to ignore heart disease. Heart disease is also expensive, costing the NHS over £500 million a year, taking up over 5000 hospital beds at any one time and resulting in the loss of 35 million working days per annum.

There are many factors linked to heart disease, including first and foremost smoking, and also heredity, high cholesterol levels, obesity and lack of exercise. Diet plays an important role and the ACE vitamins have been shown to help prevent heart disease. A recently concluded study at the University of California at Los Angeles links low levels of vitamin C to an increased risk of heart disease. Researchers found that those who consumed high levels of vitamin C had reduced death rates from heart disease. Studies over a ten-year period found that men who ate the most vitamin C had a 45 per cent lower death rate, while women had a 25 per cent lower risk. These are astonishing results and no other dietary change, including lowering high blood chlosterol with a low-fat diet, can reduce mortality by the margins seen in this study. Those in the higher intake groups were taking a total of 300 mg of vitamin C a day, compared to 50 mg at the lower end of the scale. According to nutrition researcher Dr Len Mervyn, 'Daily additional vitamin C has emerged as the simplest dietary change that a person can make to reduce the chances of heart disease.'

Two more important studies published in 1991 lend further weight to the theory that low levels of the ACE vitamins, notably vitamin E, lead to an increased risk of heart disease. In the first, investigators in Edinburgh and Switzerland looked at the relationship between heart disease and levels of vitamins A, C and E and beta-carotene. In a group of Scottish men, it showed that those with low vitamin E levels had nearly three times the risk of developing angina (severe chest pain), even after the classic heart disease factors such as high blood pressure, smoking and cholesterol levels had been taken into account. The authors, including Professor Michael Oliver, Director of the Wynn Institute in London, conclude that 'Some populations with a high incidence of coronary heart disease may benefit from eating diets rich in natural antioxidants, particularly vitamin E.'

The second report, published in the *American Journal of Clinical Nutrition*, described results from an international study sponsored by the World Health Organization. The study measured blood plasma levels of antioxidant nutrients, cholesterol levels and blood pressure in middle-aged men, selected at random in sixteen European cities. The researchers, among them Professor Fred Gey of the Institute of Biochemistry and Molecular Biology at the University of Berne, found that a low blood plasma level of vitamin E is the single most important risk factor in death from ischaemic heart disease – far more important than high cholesterol and blood pressure.

One way that vitamin E and other antioxidant nutrients work against heart disease is by neutralizing the free radicals involved in the very first symptoms. There are three main types of heart disease that can be helped by the ACE vitamins.

• Atherosclerosis, or hardening of the arteries.

- Angina, or chest pains due to insufficient blood supplies feeding the heart.
- Ischaemia, or the severe blockage of blood vessels.

Atherosclerosis

Otherwise known as the hardening of the arteries, this can begin as early as childhood. In fact, some researchers are calling for cholesterol tests for all children (available in America from the age of two onwards). Studies of 1800 Manchester children found that 60 per cent had cholesterol levels above average, which could lead to problems in later life. Atherosclerosis progresses at varying rates during adulthood, but goes undetected until complications begin. These are due to the gradual narrowing of the arteries that supply blood to our vital organs. The blood supply becomes increasingly constricted until eventually it is cut off altogether and part of our body tissue dies. High cholesterol levels are known to increase the risk of atherosclerosis, although it is not quite as simple as saying that cholesterol is the 'bad guy' of heart disease. Cholesterol is an essential substance to protect our vital organs. It is carried around the body by particles known as LCL (low-density lipoproteins) and HDL (high-density lipoproteins). Atherosclerosis begins when the LDLs dump excess cholesterol to create small patches of fat that line our artery walls. The exact mechanics of how these occur is not yet known and the question that has been puzzling scientists is exactly why this cholesterol builds up in the first place. Now research has discovered that the LDL cholesterol is oxidized, or turned rancid, and this leads to it being deposited in the arteries. It seems that once the oxidized LDL is damaged, other cells in the body are unable to recognize it. As a result it is taken up by special defence cells called macrophages that turn it into fatty foam cells which are stored in the artery walls. This leads to the development of the 'fatty streaks' which are the first stage of hardening of the arteries. These progressively prevent blood from flowing freely to the heart and, should a blood clot occur, will result in a heart attack.

One research project at the University of Kuopio in Finland examined the arteries of men with atherosclerosis. Using an ultrasound scanning machine to measure the thickness of the carotoid artery, it was shown that oxidized LDL was clearly present, and this is now thought to be the root cause of atherosclerosis. The good news is that this can largely be prevented by certain antioxidants, notably vitamin E, and the specialist Dr Mitchinson of Cambridge University describes this discovery as 'potentially momentous'. One obvious way to prevent the oxidation of LDL from happening in the first place is to make sure we have a good supply of antioxidant vitamins, the most important of which are believed to be the ACE vitamins beta-carotene, vitamin C and vitamin E. Many studies now show that the more ACE vitamins in the bloodstream, the less build-up of the arterial plaque that causes atherosclerosis.

Angina
The term 'angina' is given to an acute pain or sense of suffocation in the centre of the chest. It is usually brought on by exercise or other kinds of physical activity. Angina occurs when the heart's demand for blood exceeds the supply available, and this may be fatal. Several interesting studies indicate that the ACE vitamins can help angina patients. One of the largest projects took place in Scotland, where there is a higher than average rate of heart disease. In all, 6000 men aged between thirty-five and fifty-four were involved. As previously mentioned, researchers found that those with low levels of vitamins C and E had a significantly greater risk of angina. A further study in Australia has indicated that beta-carotene may also work against heart disease. A two-year trial using 20 mg beta-carotene daily was shown to raise levels of HDL; which is considered to be good for the heart because it transports cholesterol away from the arteries and returns it to the liver for disposal.

Ischaemia
Another serious form of heart disease is known to the

medical profession as acute myocardial ischaemia. This occurs when there is a blockage in a blood vessel. In this case, the cells that are downstream of the blockage are left dangerously short of oxygen. Although these blockages are usually temporary, the sudden restart of the blood-flow and subsequent re-oxygenation cause a burst of free radicals. This can overload our natural antioxidant defence mechanism and damage the cells of the heart. Therefore, we may be protected by having good supplies of the ACE vitamins in our bloodstream to cope with this sudden burst of free radicals. One situation where this may be especially useful is in open heart surgery. This procedure can cause tissue damage as subsequent restoration of blood and oxygen to the heart following surgery can cause a surge of free radical activity. A study reported in a specialist surgical journal showed that pre-treating a group of patients with coronary heart disease with 2000 IU vitamin E, twelve hours before surgery, prevented the significant increase in free radical levels in the blood, which is usually seen.

The role of antioxidants in heart disease suggests that, as a preventive measure, we should not only cut down on fatty foods and stop smoking, but also keep our levels of the ACE vitamins high. The theory that vitamin E, in particular, reduces heart disease appears to be borne out by major studies currently being carried out in women at the Brigham and Women's Hospital at Harvard. These were started in 1980 and, as previously mentioned in Chapter 2, involve over 87,000 nurses who filled in a detailed food and vitamin analysis to accompany their regular questionnaires. Early results in 1988 clearly showed that those who ate the most vitamin E had the least risk of heart disease. This result was due to taking vitamin E supplements as there was little or no difference in those who simply tried to eat more vitamin E-rich foods such as wheatgerm. This conclusion was published in the *New England Journal of Medicine* in June 1993.

This report also reveals that those with the highest levels of vitamin E have the most protection from heart disease, concluding: 'We observed no significant effect from vitamin E from dietary sources alone. The apparent beneficial effect of supplements was limited to use for two or more years. These data and other evidence, suggest that vitamin E supplements may reduce coronary heart disease risk.'

Professor Charles Hennekens is one of the senior researchers involved with the Harvard trial. He is cautious about the results but says:

'antioxidant vitamins are promising, but unproven, for decreasing the risk of coronary heart disease. Strictly randomized comparisons are needed – of sufficient dose and duration – and these are now underway.'

The nurses taking part in the trial are taking 50 mg beta carotene and 600 IU of natural vitamin E a day. In the next few years we should have conclusive proof as to whether vitamin supplements should be taken to prevent the risk of heart disease.

Meanwhile, there is no doubt that a wholefood, vitamin-rich diet is of great benefit for overall good health, and we should not abandon good eating habits in favour of popping pills. Dr Rudolph Riemersma, who is currently conducting trials for the British Heart Foundation, says that there is evidence that those who suffer chest pains have low levels of vitamin C, found in fresh fruits and vegetables, and low levels of vitamin E, found in vegetable oils.

Further studies show that a diet rich in fruit, vegetables, nuts and grains reduces the risk of recurring heart disease. A study of 505 patients at the Medical Hospital and Research Centre, Moradabad, India found that this diet was especially important for those who had just had a heart attack in order to increase their chances of survival. The ultimate goal of all the research being carried out into coronary heart disease is to establish a sure-fire method of prevention. Studies are now underway at Guy's and St Thomas's Hospitals in London to see if giving doses of the ACE vitamins *before* any signs of heart disease are noted will help prevent the enormous loss of life it causes.

Cancer

The Big C is another frighteningly common disease which has so far defied those in search of a cure, although we do at least know something of how the disease strikes. Cancer is a disease characterized by the excessive growth of cells and a disturbance of the cells' normal functions. All cells divide to create new ones and this process of cell division is usually kept closely under control by specific genes. Any damage to these genes by free radicals can result in the instruction for cell division being left permanently switched on. This leads to the cells rapidly multiplying out of control. Although we know how cancer can occur, it is still not clear why it affects some and not others. Unfortunately, cases of cancer are also on the increase. Although lung cancer has decreased in men by about 15 per cent in the last decade (due to giving up smoking), it increased by 20 per cent in women, who are smoking more cigarettes than ever before. Even after taking into account the increase in lung and throat cancer due to smoking, there has also been a sharp rise in other types of cancer. Data from the Swedish Cancer Registry, set up in 1958, show that cancer rates are rising across Europe. Figures reveal an increase of between a half and a third in all age groups and in both sexes. Especially worrying is the rise in cancers in children and young adults. The Swedish researchers say that the most likely reasons for the increase are environmental factors, including cancer-causing agents such as pollution. Their report states: 'Our data strongly suggest increased population exposure to carcinogens.'

In the midst of this bad news there is a glimmer of hope for the people of Europe and other nations. Encouraging epidemiological studies clearly show that many types of cancer are largely linked to diet, and in particular to the amounts of ACE vitamins eaten. The rates of cancer vary from country to country, often depending upon what foods and nutrients are eaten. For example, stomach cancer is common in Japan and low in America, whereas cases of large intestine cancer are low in Japan and high in the USA. Yet, when Japanese settle in America they soon develop the same pattern of cancers.

The biggest ever dietary survey is being co-ordinated by the International Agency for Research on Cancer (IARC) in Lyon, France. It aims to monitor around half a million people and their eating habits. Its first phase, lasting four years, focuses on the connections between diet and some of the commoner cancers such as those of the lung, colon, prostate, stomach and breast. In Britain, national organizers are recruiting some 75,000 men and women over two years. Two nutrition centres at Oxford and Cambridge are co-ordinating the British project. The Imperial Cancer Research Fund's epidemiology unit at Oxford is to recruit 50,000 subjects, while the Dunn Nutrition Unit in Cambridge will recruit 25,000 volunteers from East Anglia. Overall, this is the biggest dietary survey to date, and Europe is the ideal testing ground as each country has such a different diet. The Scots eat the most saturated fats (from meat, cream and cheese) and the least fruits and vegetables, while the Sicilians eat more monounsaturated fats (mainly from olive oil) and many more fresh fruits and vegetables.

Just as the type of food varies from Northern Europe to the Southern Mediterranean, so do the types of cancer that occur. Those living in Southern Italy, Spain and Greece are thought to be protected from many types of cancer because of the high levels of ACE vitamins that they eat. Their diet is rich in olive oil (for vitamin E), fresh fruits and vegetables (for beta-carotene and vitamin C). This trans-European study will assess the intakes of each of the ACE vitamins through detailed questionnaires and food diaries. Subjects will also give blood and urine samples for analysis. Each blood sample will be separated into four parts – plasma, serum, white cells and red blood cells – all containing certain biochemical markers which reflect the individual's state of health. For example, analysis of DNA in the samples will show how it is damaged following attack by free radicals.

The cancer connection

Beta-carotene: In 1981, a landmark article was published in the scientific journal *Nature*, which suggested that eating more beta-carotene might substantially reduce the risk of developing cancer. This was based on the results of a number of trials that had taken place around the world. One of the first to look at levels of beta-carotene in the diet took place in Chicago between 1957 and 1969. In this case, 2000 workers at the Western Electric Company were assessed over a ten-year period. They were examined annually until 1969 when it was discovered that those who ate the most vegetables, fruit and soup had the lowest levels of cancer. These foods are among the best sources of beta-carotene.

Vitamin C: One of the most important documents to link vitamin C with cancer prevention was recently published by Professor Gladys Block at the National Cancer Institute in the USA. Her paper, entitled 'Vitamin C and cancer prevention; the epidemiologic evidence', cites forty-six different studies looking at the role of vitamin C in preventing cancer. In thirty-three of these, researchers found a link between high levels of vitamin C and low levels of cancer. Of a further twenty-one studies which looked at the amount of fruit eaten in the diet, all showed a positive effect against cancer. Fruit, of course, is our richest food source of vitamin C.

Vitamin E: There have been many studies over the last decade to show that vitamin E reduced the incidence of cancer in animals, and these have been backed by human epidemiological research. In four large-scale studies involving around 85,000 people in Finland, a reduced risk of cancers was shown in those with higher vitamin E levels, or a greater cancer risk in those with low supplies. Some of this data shows quite clearly that those with low levels of vitamin E in their bloodstream are at a much greater risk of diseases such as breast cancer. Further studies are currently underway, but researchers are suggesting that the protection comes from vitamin E preserving the fat-filled membrane that surrounds all our cells.

The ACE vitamin team: During the last decade, vast resources have been channelled into research which suggests that beta-carotene, together with vitamins C and E, can help prevent some types of cancer. It is difficult to isolate any one of these nutrients as being the most important as they all interact with each other. For example, vitamin E is strengthened by vitamin C, while the action of beta-carotene is enhanced by vitamin E. Scientists are now investigating the possibility of an 'anti-cancer cocktail' that contains each of the ACE vitamins for future cancer prevention.

Lung cancer

Lung cancer is the biggest killer of all cancers and can be largely prevented by stopping smoking and not breathing in others' cigarette smoke. The act of breathing in poisonous air in the form of tobacco smoke force-feeds the body with free radicals and dramatically reduces levels of ACE vitamins. A Norwegian study in 1975 originally sparked the speculation that one of the ACE vitamins could protect against lung cancer. At the time, the researchers did not connect beta-carotene with these results but said they believed the protective factor was vitamin A or 'closely related dietary factors'. This led to more research being carried out that pin-pointed beta-carotene as the active nutrient, not vitamin A itself. Studies were set up to examine the plasma of volunteers before and after cancer struck. Blood samples from cancer-free volunteers were collected and frozen. All cases of subsequent cancer were recorded and it was found that those who developed lung cancer had lower levels of beta-carotene in their blood sample than those who remained free from the disease. Further research soon followed and in 1971, the ACE vitamins were analysed again while blood samples from 6800 men living on the island of Oahu in Hawaii were examined. Ten years later, researchers found that there was a strong association between low-serum beta-carotene levels and the risk of lung cancer. In fact, those with the lowest levels were more than three times as likely to die from the disease. Further work with volunteers from pharmaceutical companies in Basel, Switzerland, found that of 2974 subjects, 204 died of cancer. Researchers discovered that these victims had signficantly lower levels of beta-carotene than the survivors. This risk was especially raised for lung cancer, which claimed sixty-eight lives.

Smokers were again targeted in the 1980's for a research project carried out at St Bartholomew's Hospital Medical School in London, involving 22,000 men aged between thirty-five and sixty-four. The concentration of beta-carotene was measured in 271 of these men who subsequently developed lung cancer. Two controls were selected for each of the subjects matched on age, number of cigarettes smoked, etc. Heavy smokers had the lowest beta-carotene levels and, interestingly, the study found that the effect was present 'five or more years *before* the diagnosis of cancer'. This means that in the future, a simple blood test could determine our risk of developing this disease. The medical world has become so excited at the prospect of vitamins protecting against cancer that more major trials are currently underway. One on-going project at Harvard Medical School is studying cancer in all parts of the body and links with the amount of beta-carotene eaten. This study began in 1982 with the participation of 22,000 male doctors between the ages of forty and eighty-four, all of whom were healthy and not 'at risk' from any known disorder. The physicians are currently taking 50 mg of beta carotene every other day and the results of this trial in 1995 will be of major significance. A further study of 29,000 male smokers in Finland has been divided into four groups: respectively taking supplements with beta-carotene, vitamin E, a combination of the two and a placebo. This long-term study began in 1984 and is studying the incidence of cancer (especially lung cancer) and coronary heart disease.

Vitamin E has also been shown to play a protective role in the case of lung cancer. A study of more than 25,000 people in Maryland showed that those with the least beta-carotene and vitamin E in their blood were at greatest risk of this disease. In this case, low levels of vitamin E meant their likelihood of lung cancer was more than doubled. Most of the studies since then have focused on beta-carotene and vitamin E as preventing lung cancer, but vitamin C also plays a role. A study carried out in the Netherlands looked at the importance of vitamin C-rich foods, such as oranges, in the diet of smokers. Those with the lowest levels of vitamin C were found to have the highest risk of lung cancer. Professor Gladys Block has since looked at eleven such nutrition studies which specifically mention vitamin C. She concludes that 'the recent data reported suggests an important protective effect of vitamin C intake. The role of vitamin C not only as an antioxidant and free radical scavenger in its own right, but also in enhancing the action of vitamin E is well established.' In other words, vitamin C is needed to support the action of vitamin E. All in all, the evidence now exists to show that each of the three ACE vitamins may give significant protection against lung cancer.

Stomach cancer

Stomach and bowel cancers kill around 30,000 men and women in Britain each year, a figure that is second only to lung cancer. Because our stomach, digestive tract and colon are in constant contact with the food we eat, researchers have been studying the effect of our diet on these types of cancer. An Italian study involving over 2000 volunteers found that there was a five-fold difference in risk between those with high vitamin C and vitamin E intake and low protein and nitrite intake. This would indicate that cutting down on high-protein foods such as meat and dairy produce and any smoked foods that contain nitrites is a sensible precaution against avoid stomach cancer. The World Cancer Research Fund issues dietary guidelines to lower your risk of cancer. To help stop cancer before it starts:

1. Eat less fat and fewer fatty foods.
2. Eat more fruit, vegetables and wholegrain cereals.

3. Eat fewer salt-cured, salt-pickled and smoked foods containing nitrites.
4. Drink less alcohol.
5. Eat far more fibre.

Further studies have also shown that those with stomach and colon cancer have lower levels of the ACE vitamins. Cancers of the colon and rectum are surprisingly common and are thought to be due to pre-cancerous polyps called ademonas. Researchers at the University of Bologna, Italy examined the effects of six months' treatment with a combination of vitamins A (not beta-carotene this time), C and E, at daily doses of 30,000 IU, 100 mg and 70 mg respectively, on the growth of these ademonas. Those receiving the vitamins showed a decrease in cell proliferation compared to the control-patients. The authors conclude 'These findings suggest that vitamin A, C and E supplementation is effective in reducing abnormalities in cell kinetics that may indicate a pre-cancerous condition.' A further compilation of five studies of colorectal cancer conducted in Finland, Hawaii, Maryland, Basel and London shows that those with the highest levels of vitamin E tend to have the lowest risks of colorectal cancer.

Cervical cancer
American Indian women living in the south-western USA have an unusually high risk of cervical cancer, although it is not understood why. Known risk factors such as smoking, early sexual intercourse, a history of sexually transmitted diseases or infection with the *apailloma* virus are all relatively uncommon. There is some evidence to suggest that cervical cancer is linked to diet and researchers at the University of New Mexico found that these women with cervical cancer also had low levels of vitamin C and folic acid (one of the B-complex vitamins). A further American study linked low levels of beta-carotene and vitamin C with a high risk of cervical cancer. In this case, women who ate the fewest dark green or yellow vegetables, such

as cabbage, carrots and peppers, and who drank the least fruit juice were at greatest risk. All these foods are excellent sources of beta-carotene and vitamin C. Vitamin E has also been shown to play a protective role. Again, American studies report that a high intake of vitamin E is associated with a significantly lower risk of cervical cancer.

Oral cancer

There have been several trials that demonstrate the ability of beta-carotene to reverse oral leukoplakia. These are white patches inside the mouth caused by smoking or alcohol that can become malignant. We know that vitamin A is essential to keep the mucous membranes inside the mouth healthy, but too much vitamin A can cause problems. Therefore, researchers turned to beta-carotene, the safe vegetable form of vitamin A, to see if this had a similar effect. A review in the *International Journal of Cancer* in 1986 states: 'A series of studies demonstrated that beta-carotene alone or in combination with vitamin A can decrease the incidence of micronucleated cells in exfoliated micronucleated cells (these probably indicated genotoxic damage produced by carcinogens) from populations at risk of oral cancer.' The following study was carried out in India where oral lesions are common due to the habit of chewing betel nuts, which are known to cause cancer. In this case, the three groups were treated with 180 mg beta-carotene, 180 mg beta-carotene plus vitamin A 30 mg or a placebo (sugar pill). After six months of treatment, 15 per cent of the patients in group one and 27.5 per cent of the patients in group two, compared to just 3 per cent in the third group, had complete remission of their disease. Interestingly, the recurrence of new tumours was also strongly inhibited, indicating that beta-carotene and vitamin A may also have a protective effect. A further study published in the *Journal of Clinical Oncology* in 1990 noted that oral cancer patients who were given a daily 30 mg dose of beta-carotene for three to six months responded positively in over 70 per cent of cases. There were no side-effects and the author concluded: 'Beta-carotene fulfils all the criteria for a suitable chemopreventive agent in that it is non-toxic, cheap and is a nutrient.'

One of the most recent studies looked at the role of all the ACE vitamins in preventing oral and pharyngeal cancer. This research, conducted in New Jersey, Atlanta, Los Angeles and Santa Clara and San Mateo counties in California, involved 1114 patients with oral cancer compared to 1268 people without the disease. Each patient was matched with a healthy subject living in the same area, of the same age, race and sex. They were all questioned about the vitamin supplements they took, but not the doses. Researchers analysed major risk factors such as smoking and alcohol consumption and found that those who took supplements of the individual beta-carotene, vitamin C and vitamin E had a lower risk of oral cancer than those who did not. Researchers were staggered to find that those who regularly took vitamin E supplements halved their risk of oral cancer. This was the first study to demonstrate a protective effect of vitamin E against oral cancer in humans and the authors concluded: 'Single-entity vitamin E supplements such as those found to be protective in this study generally contain 100 IU or more of the vitamin. The lack of effect of multi-vitamins and dietary vitamin E may reflect the low doses of vitamin E obtained from these sources. Thus the findings of this study suggest that vitamin E doses substantially higher than the current recommendations are needed to reduce oral cancer risk.'

Breast cancer
One of the most impressive findings has linked low levels of vitamin E with a higher risk of breast cancer. Researchers in Finland found that when vitamin E was measured from stored blood serum samples during an eight-year period, those with the lowest levels had the greatest chance of developing breast cancer. In fact, those with the least vitamin E and selenium in their bloodstream had a ten-fold higher risk of breast cancer. According to the researchers, these results suggest that low-serum vitamin E

concentration can predict cancer development in women. In a follow-up study in the UK, low levels of vitamin E were related to a significantly higher risk of subsequent breast cancer. In this case, 5000 women in Guernsey aged between twenty-eight and seventy-five years gave a blood sample which was then frozen. Women who went on to develop breast cancer were then involved in the study. The frozen blood plasma samples were retrieved and compared to two other control samples frozen at the same time. The samples from the women with breast cancer were matched as closely as possible to other women of the same age, menstrual cycle and family history of breast cancer. It was found that women who had the lowest levels of vitamin E had five times the risk of developing breast cancer. Beta-carotene levels also tended to be lower in the women who went on to get breast cancer. Further studies in the USA show that low beta-carotene levels do indeed increase the chance of developing breast cancer. A case-control study compared plasma levels of beta-carotene and vitamin A in eighty-three patients with breast cancer and 113 women without the disease. Those with the lowest beta-carotene levels were seen as having the greatest risk of breast cancer. No such relationship has been recorded with vitamin A. This indicates that it is the antioxidant action of beta-carotene and vitamin E that is giving women protection from this deadly disease.

Skin cancer

Skin cancer is the fastest-growing cancer in Britain and is increasing at an alarming rate. This is one reason why scientists are now looking at the role the ACE vitamins play in helping to prevent this disease. Vitamin E has long been used in skin creams to delay the signs of wrinkles, but it may also help prevent skin cancer. In a study where mice were rubbed with vitamin E three times a week for three weeks before exposure to ultra-violet radiation (the same as in sunshine), it cut the incidence of skin cancer by half. One reason for this could be that sunlight reduces Langerhan's cells, which are part of the skin's natural defence system. Using vitamin E directly on the skin can give these important cells an additional layer of protection. This added safety factor may also help guard against skin disorders such as cold sores caused by the herpes simplex virus, which flourish when the immune system is under attack. In addition, vitamin E has been shown to be effective at preventing mild sunburn when rubbed on the skin. In fact, it is such an effective skin shield that it can be given a low SPF (sun protection factor), similar to those seen on bottles of sunscreen. This is because vitamin E protects the skin against free radical skin damage caused by ultra-violet light, although it is also necessary to protect the skin with an additional sunblock when outside in strong sunlight.

Epilepsy

As with cancers, the numbers of people with epilepsy is on the increase and as yet there is no cure. The term 'epilepsy' covers a range of brain disorders characterized by sudden, recurrent attacks. Having epilepsy does not mean permanent brain damage, but for many it means living in constant fear of another convulsive seizure. Some kinds of epilepsy can be controlled, but not cured, by drugs. Other variations of the disorder remain unresponsive. Vitamin E has been shown to help those whose epilepsy does not respond to drug treatment. One trial at the neurology department of the Sonoma Developmental Centre in California has shown that high doses of vitamin E reduced the frequency and severity of epileptic fits. Fifty-two patients between the ages of five and sixty-two were tested. All the volunteers had moderate to severe epilepsy, which did not respond well to conventional medications. Over the course of a year, those taking the vitamin E supplements recorded a 32 per cent reduction in the number of their seizures. Dr Anne Hom, who was in charge of the study, concluded: 'Our research suggests that supplementation with natural vitamin E has positive implications for improvement in quality of life as well as the cost of care for epileptic patients.'

Fertility

Vitamin E has been strongly linked to fertility ever since it was established that low levels caused sterility in animals. Since then, researchers have been looking to see if there is the same connection in humans. Dr Aitken of the Medical Research Council's reproductive biology unit in Edinburgh has found that the sperm in some infertile men produce up to forty times the normal level of hydrogen peroxide. 'This makes the men infertile by oxidizing crucial cell membrane fats in the sperm and preventing fusion with the egg. We hope that the antioxidant activity of vitamin E will counteract this.' Trials are currently underway to prove this theory. Meanwhile, Dr Aitken's findings are a major advance as sperm defects are the most common cause of infertility in couples.

A clear link between low levels of vitamin C and genetically damaged sperm has been established in a study by Dr Bruce Ames of the University of California in Los Angeles. In this case, the low levels of vitamin C were caused by cigarette smoking, which wipes out vitamin C in the body. Dr Ames' study showed that low levels of vitamin C in fathers due to smoking cause early death and genetic defects in their children. No such connection could be made with their mothers. Dr Ames surveyed 15,000 children born between 1959 and 1966. His team of researchers found that the children of men who smoked more than twenty cigarettes a day were twice as likely to suffer birth defects, such as harelip and heart problems, as the children of non-smokers. Leukaemia and cancer of the lymph nodes were twice as common among the children of men who had smoked in the year before their children were born. Brain cancer was also 40 per cent more common. Dr Ames says: 'I'm already convinced that a good proportion of the birth defects and child cancers are coming from male smokers.' However, the problem is even more serious as smoking damages DNA by oxidation and so causes genetic damage that can be inherited. Dr Ames has warned that men who smoke are risking damage to their sperm, 'an effect that will reverberate down the generations'. Men who smoke may be harming not only their children, but also their grandchildren and great-grandchildren. According to Dr Ames, eating more of the ACE vitamins in the diet will help lower the risk of genetic damage by reducing the 'oxidative lesions' at points along the DNA molecule. A diet rich in vitamin C can reduce the levels of oxidative damage in sperm cells by 50 to 75 per cent. Dr Ames has since called for the US government to increase its recommended daily allowance (RDA) for vitamin C and to fund more research into exactly how much is needed to protect the cells of future generations.

Pollution

A further threat to all future generations around the world is global pollution. Both the World Health Organization and the US Environmental Protection Agency rank smog as the most dangerous threat to both animal and plant life. Unfortunately, most of Europe is breathing in levels of pollutants that far exceed the recommended guidelines. Increasing evidence suggests that many of the minor lung irritations that occur today as a result of pollution will lead to an epidemic of chronic disorders in the future.

The most important pollutant in smog is ground-level ozone. This chemical is produced in the atmosphere as sunlight mixes with car fumes and industrial pollution, and is most common in cities and other areas of urban development. During the summer months, it is not uncommon for popular holiday areas such as London, East Anglia, North Yorkshire, Cumbria and Devon regularly to exceed the safety guidelines for ozone concentrations in the air. Ozone is formed high above the earth and covers the stratosphere like a protective blanket. Its role there is to filter out the damaging sun's rays that would destroy life on earth if allowed to slip through. This is why the threat of a dramatically decreasing ozone layer is so worrying. While we need plenty of ozone overhead, it is not protective at ground level. Ozone is one of the most toxic substances on earth. It is an oxidant, meaning that it can form free radicals in the body. Even tiny quantities of ozone at around 0.3 parts per million produces emphysema (breathlessness) and other breathing difficulties, and attack our immune system. Protecting ourselves with doses of antioxidant vitamins would therefore seem to be a sensible precaution against its effects.

Professor William Pryor is the director of the Biodynamics Institute at Louisiana State University. He has made a life-long study of the effects of pollution and is a world authority on the subject of ozone damage. His work *in vitro* and with animals indicates that vitamin E protects against the damage caused by ozone. When mice are exposed to ozone their reserves of vitamin E are moved from stores in the spleen to the lungs. This indicates that the body uses vitamin E to defend itself. Leading researchers are notoriously cautious when it comes to committing themselves, but Professor Pryor goes as far as saying, 'We cannot say with certainty that vitamin E will protect the human body, but the data strongly suggests that it does.'

Evidence is also mounting that vitamin C is helpful in guarding against the ill-effects of inhaling nitrogen dioxide and sulphur dioxide, both of which are increasing in the air we breathe. Figures published by the Department of the Environment show that nitrogen oxides from traffic have already risen by a staggering 73 per cent since 1981, and studies have linked this with the sharp increase in asthma and possibly even hay fever. This is worrying news, as the Department of the Environment also predicts that traffic will increase by as much as 140 per cent by the year 2025. Many of these emissions come from diesel trucks and cars which produce three times as much nitrogen dioxide as petrol cars fitted with catalytic converters.

Nitrogen dioxide and sulphur dioxide are not only

present in the air outside but can also pose a problem in the home. Adults and children who regularly breathe the fumes given off by gas stoves have been found to be more at risk from respiratory infections. Professional cooks should note Professor Pryor's comments that some gas stoves produce fumes similar to tobacco smoke. However Dr Bob Harris from British Gas explains that the amount of sulphur oxides given off is very low, and only found in the safety odour added to gas to enable it to be detected. The level of nitrogen dioxide emissions from a gas hob also depends on the temperature and intensity of the flame – the hotter it is, the more is given off. Many more noxious emissions may come from a hot gas fire than a stove.

Vitamin C may help prevent the damage caused by both nitrogen dioxide and sulphur dioxide. One way this vitamin appears to work is by boosting our tolerance to histamine and prevent allergic reactions. Until a time when we can enjoy a smog-free environment, those living in urban areas could consider taking a daily supplement of vitamins C and E to protect themselves against the side-effects of pollution. This is an especially important consideration for children who risk damage to their fundamental growth.

A report by the National Children's Bureau in March 1993 said that 'children are hit harder by pollution because they are smaller, still developing and physiologically immature. Generally their bodies are quicker to absorb toxic substances and slower to eliminate them. Children are therefore particularly badly affected by contaminated air, drinking water, land and beaches. The well-being of children in the UK is adversely affected by environmental factors which harm their health or stunt their development.'

According to Professor Daniel Menzel at the Department of Community and Environmental Medicine, University of California, 'The slow, long-term effects of continuing exposure to air pollution on the development of the lung also suggests that children should be provided protection by supplementation.'

Premature Babies

Vitamins play an important role in the development of all babies and small children, but for premature babies they may be life-saving. Before a baby is born it relies solely on its mother for regular supplies of nutrients. These are passed to the unborn child via the mother's bloodstream, which is why it is so important for a pregnant woman to watch her diet and eat well (there is more about this in the following chapter). However, recent research has revealed that some nutrients are not passed on to the baby until around the last stage of pregnancy. These include certain essential fatty acids that are involved in brain development, and also vitamin E. For most babies who are born on time this does not present a problem. But for a premature baby this could mean the difference between life or death. Because vitamin E does not cross over the placental barrier to the baby until the thirty-sixth week of pregnancy (four weeks before the child is due), a prematurely born baby will not have its own reserves of vitamin E. In addition, as soon as a pre-term baby is born it is usually placed in an incubator and given very necessary additional oxygen. As we now know, oxygen is the prime source of free radicals and such a sudden exposure is likely to create a surge of these in the infant, who is lacking the vitamin E needed to combat this imbalance of free radical activity. Research carried out by Dr Catherine Rice-Evans, director of the Free Radical Research Group, looked at pre-term babies between twenty-five and twenty-nine weeks' gestation. These were all found to have significantly low levels of vitamin E, as the vitamin had not been passed on from their mothers. Tests were carried out by taking blood samples from the umbilical cord just after the babies were delivered. Further blood samples were obtained from the standard 'heel prick' or Guthrie test which is routinely carried out when a baby is five days old. From these tests it is possible to see that babies born with higher levels of vitamin E in their bloodstream are better protected against free radical cell damage. The study concludes that 'monitoring maternal antioxidant levels during pregnancy where indicated may also be ultimately beneficial to the neonate'.

In the future, vitamin E may join forces with folic acid and iron as a nutrient that should be supplemented during pregnancy. These nutrients play an important role in protecting the health and development of the unborn child. We already know that folic acid should be taken during the early stages of pregnancy to prevent spina bifida. This is so important that the British government now advises *all* women who might have even the slightest chance of becoming pregnant to take additional folic acid which will protect the foetus in its first few weeks of life. Timing is especially important here, as the neural tube closes at around the fourth week, before many women even realise they are pregnant. An additional study reported in the *British Medical Journal* in June 1993 found that multivitamin supplements taken around the time of conception also reduced the risk of major congenital abnormalities. Researchers in Budapest looked at over 4000 pregnancies and found that the rate of birth defects such as cleft palates, limb and organ deficiencies and heart problems was significantly lower among women taking a multivitamin supplement. It is certainly clear that eating a well-balanced diet that includes foods rich in beta-carotene, vitamins C and E will help give babies the best start in life and may protect them from life-long disorders.

5
ACE PLAN IN ACTION!

Putting the ACE Plan into action for life-long healthy living is as easy as learning your A.C.E. There are just two steps to take to ensure your ACE Plan protection:

1. Reduce your exposure to free radicals.
2. Boost your levels of the ACE vitamins.

Sounds easy? It is!

The free radical factor

The first step to better health and improved well-being is to reduce your risk of internal cell damage by producing too many free radicals. A few are needed by the body to fight bacteria and for other important processes, but a surplus supply soon starts to destroy cells within the system. As we have seen, excessive action of free radicals has a wide-ranging destructive effect inside the body. Free radicals have been linked to just about every degenerative disease, including arthritis, cancer, cataracts, coronary heart disease, epilepsy and Parkinson's disease as well as skin wrinkling. By avoiding the main sources of free radicals we will automatically reduce our risk of contracting such disorders.

Here's how to reduce your risk of free radical damage:

ACE Plan Don'ts:

1. Don't smoke! Not even one cigarette – not ever! Cigarette smoking is a prime source of free radicals within the body.
2. Avoid passive smoking – who wants to breathe in free radicals? Make your home and office a smoke-free zone.
3. Protect yourself from pollution: avoid traffic jams and the build-up of toxic exhaust fumes whenever possible, escape to the countryside to take in lungfuls of fresh air when you can, invest in a portable air purifier to screen out any harmful pollutants in the air at home and work.
4. If you have a choice, move to a less urban environment where there are no obvious sources of pollution, such as main roads, foundries, chemical works, etc.
5. Don't eat foods containing nitrites. These cancer-causing agents increase free radical activity. Check the labels on all smoked foods before buying.
6. Don't drink water with a high concentration of nitrates. Check with your water authority on local nitrate levels in your drinking water. If in doubt, drink bottled water with a low nitrate content (check the label and compare brands) or use an inexpensive jug water filter.
7. Don't expose yourself to more radiation than you need to. Ask your doctor or dentist if that X-ray is absolutely essential.
8. Don't expose your skin to strong sunshine. Ultraviolet light dramatically increases free radical activity in the skin, leading to wrinkles and potential problems such as skin cancer.

The ACE Vitamins

The second stage to improved health and vitality is to ensure a good level of nutrition, including the all-important ACE vitamins: beta-carotene, vitamin C and vitamin E. All are antioxidants, meaning they fight against the oxidation caused by free radicals. All help protect our cells and prevent the damage and destruction triggered by free radical activity. The ACE Plan guidelines for healthy eating are remarkably simple: focus on fruit, vegetables and whole grains to boost your levels of beta-carotene, vitamin C and vitamin E. Avoid processed, refined foods that have been stripped of their precious nutrients. Here's how to maximize your levels of ACE vitamins and prevent free radical cell damage:

ACE Plan Do's

1. Do watch what you eat – read labels, check vitamin levels and be aware of the foods your family is eating.
2. Do increase the amount of fruit and vegetables every member of the family eats. The World health Organisation advises us to eat 400 g (nearly 1 lb) of fruit and vegetables (excluding potatoes) every day. The most recent American guidelines advise a staggering five to nine portions each day! (A portion is an amount that would roughly fill a teacup.)
3. Do increase your level of wholegrain cereals. Look for the words 'whole' on packaged foods, such as wholewheat pasta and wholemeal bread.
4. Do avoid drinking excessive amounts of alcohol. Excess alcohol encourages free radical activity.
5. Do cover up and protect the skin against the free radicals produced by strong sunshine by wearing long sleeves and a wide-brimmed hat. If you're worried about wrinkles, always use a sunblock on top of your usual moisturizer – even on cloudy days.
6. Do choose a suncream that has the word 'block' on the label. Sunblock is far more effective at protecting the skin than sunscreen.

7. Do remain active and take regular exercise, but consider taking a supplement of vitamin E when working the body hard. This helps reduce the free radical damage by breathing in additional oxygen.
8. Do consider whether you, or members of your family, need to top up daily levels of the ACE vitamins with a regular supplement.

Supplements for a radical difference

For many years we have been told by nutritionists and doctors that if we eat a 'well-balanced diet' we do not need to take vitamin supplements. However, the research that has been documented in the ACE Plan reveals that this may not be the case. The official line of the government and organizations such as the Health Education Authority still maintains that if we eat a varied diet we do not need to take supplements. However, this guideline was drawn up long before the recent research into antioxidants became known. In the past, advice for taking vitamins and minerals has been based on a recommended daily allowance (RDA). This quantity is partly based on the amount of a nutrient necessary to prevent deficiency diseases. For example, vitamin C is needed to prevent scurvy, vitamin B1 to prevent beri beri and vitamin D to prevent rickets. What we do not yet know is by how much these need to be increased to take into account the new-found antioxidant properties of some nutrients. According to Anthony Diplock, Professor of Biochemistry at Guy's Medical School, 'The current recommendations for vitamin E and other antioxidants are inconsistent with actual human requirements for optimal nutrition.'

Yet it is not possible to define RDAs for the antioxidant action of the ACE vitamins because there are no direct deficiency diseases involved. You don't instantly die from a shortage of vitamin E, although the long-term health implications may be serious. Likewise, supplements of vitamin E should not be seen as a quick-fix, but thought of as part of a long-term health strategy. We are well aware of the minimum quantities of some vitamins needed to

ACE VITAMINS CAN HELP PREVENT DISEASE

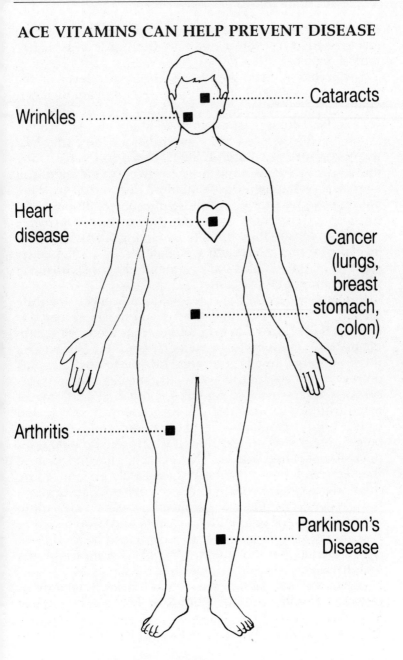

prevent deficiency diseases, but what are the optimum levels needed to protect our cells from an excess of free radical activity?

The million-dollar question is this: what level of the ACE vitamins should we be receiving to prevent degenerative disease? Can we get enough from our diet, or should we all be taking a supplement? Many of the studies involving disorders such as heart disease have involved quantities such as vitamin E 400 IU (294 mg of natural vitamin E) daily. But does this necessarily mean we should all start swallowing high-dose capsules? Unfortunately, there are no obvious answers to these questions, although the research is currently underway to produce conclusive findings. Meanwhile, foods containing naturally high levels of vitamins have always been thought to be better healthwise than taking a supplement. However, this may not necessarily be the case.

Researchers from the US National Cancer Institute carried out a control trial where volunteers received a defined daily dose of beta-carotene from foods, or a supplement containing solely beta-carotene. For six weeks, the testers ate a strictly controlled low-carotenoid diet plus daily doses of one of the test foods, such as carrots, broccoli or tomato juice, or capsules containing 12-30 mg of beta-carotene, or a control placebo. The main conclusion of this study was that 'The plasma response to purified beta-carotene was greater than it was to similar quantities of carotenoids from foods.' The difference may be because the beta-carotene in foods is not as readily assimilated by the body because of differences in intestinal absorption. Researchers conclude that because it would be difficult to eat much greater quantities of carrots and broccoli every day, it may be more effective to recommend beta-carotene supplements than to attempt major alterations to the nation's diet.

There are also good reasons for taking vitamin E capsules. Studies recently published in the *New England Journal of Medicine* have shown that the protective effect of vitamin E against heart disease was not derived from vitamin E in the diet, but from taking vitamin E supplements. Another factor is that vitamin E is not widely available in the foods we eat. It can be found in wholemeal bread, wheatgerm, unrefined cooking oils (where it has not been removed by the refining process), nuts and seeds, but a small sprinkling of sunflower seeds or wheatgerm on your breakfast cereal is not going to contribute a great deal to your levels of vitamin E: you would need to eat 450 g (1 lb) of sunflower seeds, more than 2.5 kg (5 lb) of wheatgerm or drink over 2 litres (4 pints) of corn oil a day to achieve the same intake of vitamin E found in a common 400 IU capsule supplement. In addition, many of the foods containing vitamin E, such as asparagus and avocados, are more expensive than other foods and therefore infrequent purchases.

Senior researchers around the world are now breaking the habit of a life-time and speaking in terms of recommending ACE vitamin supplements to promote better health. Speaking at a conference in Baltimore in April 1993, Gladys Block, Professor of Public Health Nutrition, University of California at Berkeley, said: 'In the context of our escalating health care costs, we need to prevent cancer and other diseases. There's ample evidence that nutrients can help do this.' She added: 'Policymakers should back away from the position that you shouldn't take supplements. Antioxidant supplement use in disease prevention is inexpensive insurance. We must look at nutrition with a new perspective. In the US, for example, only 9 per cent of the population on any given day has five servings of fruit and vegetables. It is a public health mistake to limit our efforts to fruit and vegetables and tell people not to take supplements. Fortification and supplementation also should be legitimate parts of our public health armoury.'

Many health-watchers are convinced that it is only a matter of time before guidelines are introduced to recommend that every man, woman and child takes a daily supplement of the ACE vitamins. Professor Pryor of Louisiana State University believes that the USA is only about eight years away from making a public health statement that vitamin E supplements should be taken on a daily basis for the prevention of heart disease. Professor Diplock also believes that the day for recommending daily supplements on a national scale will come 'sooner, rather than later, in the interim period before the results of intervention studies are available early in the next century.'

ACE Eating

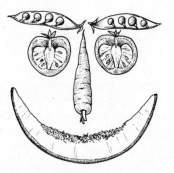

One reason why the role of supplements is assuming a greater importance is that the pattern of British eating habits has changed considerably over recent years. More women (and men) are combining a career with looking after a family. Increasing work pressures and lifestyle stresses mean that many of us are working harder and the pace of life is more hectic than ever. This can make mealtimes rushed and often shortens the amount of preparation time available for shopping and cooking. Formal family meals have been largely replaced with eating on the run, snack foods and eating out. For children, cooked school meals which were planned to give a balance of nutrients have been commonly replaced with packed lunches or self-selection cafeteria meals. Those of us who are at work all day are more likely to opt for a sandwich or a fast-food snack than a full meal. The traditional cooked breakfast at home is also a dim and distant memory for most of us. This is not such a bad thing when you consider its high fat content, but it does mean that some are tempted to skip breakfast altogether and leave home with an empty stomach. By not eating breakfast we are missing a significant source of the ACE vitamins in the form of fruit juice, fresh fruit, wholemeal toast and wholegrain cereals. By the evening, many of us are just too tired to cook. The rise in convenience and pre-prepared foods has been astronomic in recent years. Those returning home from a hard day's work are far more likely to tuck into a frozen-cum-microwaved meal than anything that has been freshly prepared. And while the more expensive convenience foods contain good levels of nutrients, many others are high in fat, salt and sugar – and low in the ACE vitamins.

The culmination of these drastic social changes over the decade has led to more people making their own choices about what they eat, and choosing processed foods that are quick and easy to prepare. This is especially true of the younger generation, many of whom will admit to being unable to cook a meal from scratch. So what do all these changes in the nation's diet actually mean in health terms? According to Professor Diplock, 'Of all the things that happens to our foods, I think processing is one of the biggest problems. Natural levels of antioxidants may be altered and there are consequences also in cooking because the antioxidants are not protected.' Professor Diplock stresses that we must all make sure our diet is high in the ACE vitamins, not just temporarily, but for the rest of our life.

A Baby's Best Start
Today's new mothers are bombarded with different dietary advice for their babies, but one thing is clear: you're never too young to start the healthy eating guidelines outlined in the ACE Plan. Having two children under the age of three, I am especially aware of the importance of vitamins, minerals and other essential nutrients that are needed to build healthy bodies.

PREMATURE BABIES
Premature babies have special needs. If your baby is born prematurely or has a low birth weight, extra vitamins may be necessary. These may be added to breast-milk that has been expressed by the mother, or added to special formula feeds. Most doctors are aware of this and it is important to discuss with your paediatrician if this may be necessary. According to researcher Dr Catherine Rice-Evans, 'Doctors keep premature babies alive these days at incredibly low birth weights. In order to keep the babies alive they need high concentrations of oxygen, which unfortunately are a source of free radicals. Therefore a premature baby needs all the antioxidants available. Premature babies don't have any vitamin E in their bloodstream because this doesn't cross to the placenta until the third trimester. For these reasons it is very important for the mother to have a good intake of antioxidant vitamins before and during the pregnancy, as well as while breast-feeding.' Unfortunately, many premature babies are not breast-fed because the mother's milk dries up while the infant is in an incubator. If your baby is born prematurely, it is worth keeping your supply of breast-milk going by expressing with a portable pump. The expressed milk can either be fed to a pre-term baby or frozen for later use. You will then be able to continue breast-feeding when your baby is discharged from hospital.

BABY MILKS
As soon as babies are born, they become dependent on the outside world for all their nutritional needs. Instead of receiving an automatic flow of nutrients from their mother's bloodstream, they must obtain them either from breast-milk or formula feeds. As everyone knows, breast is best. This is because it contains antibodies, human growth factors, and more nutrients than formula milks. For this reason, the government's Health of the Nation Green Paper aims to have 75 per cent of all new mothers breast-feeding by the year 2000. Breast-milk contains beta-carotene and selenium (both antioxidant nutrients) as well as

the essential fatty acids GLA, DHA and EPA. None of these is added to off-the-shelf milks, although traces of selenium and some of the essential fatty acids may be present in powdered cow's milk. A 1991 EC directive on formula milks states that beta-carotene can be safely added to feeds, but as yet no British brands do this. A breast-fed baby also receives more vitamin C and vitamin E, provided that the mother is eating good sources of these, such as fruits, vegetables and whole grains, or taking a daily supplement. A great deal of research is currently underway to determine what difference these nutrients make early in life as the child develops. Studies have been published in *The Lancet* to show that babies who are breast-fed grow up to be marginally more intelligent than formula-fed babies. Researchers at the Medical Research Council's Dunn Nutrition Unit in Cambridge found that premature babies who had been fed their mother's milk by tube had, by the time they reached seven or eight years of age, significantly higher IQ's than those who were given formula feeds. This may be connected in some way to the additional levels of the ACE vitamins or the essential fatty acids that the children received.

We also know that new-borns are better protected against infections by the powerful antibodies present in breast-milk. The first milk that comes from the breast is called colostrum. This takes over where the placenta left off and provides the new-born baby with a very special milk. Colostrum is low in fat and carbohydrates, and high in protein. It is also a rich source of vitamin E. Colostrum is extremely easy for a new-born to digest and acts as an instant pick-me-up after the experience of being born into the world. For many years, the extraordinary properties of colostrum were largely ignored. However, we now know that it is loaded with living cells that go to the infant's defence against many potentially harmful disorders. In particular, colostrum contains protective white cells called leucocytes. These white cells are also found in blood and are the body's main line of defence against infections, killing off invading bacteria and viruses. There are as many white cells in colostrum as there in our bloodstream and, like blood, colostrum is a living liquid. Even if a mother decides not to breast-feed, it is important that her baby receives its supply of colostrum. The concentration of antibodies is greatest in the few hours after birth, so it is well worth putting the baby to the breast as soon as possible, and rejecting any other drinks such as glucose, water or formula milk that may be offered. After a few days, a richer, creamier milk replaces the colostrum and for forty-eight hours the new mum has a bust to rival Dolly Parton's. This soon settles down and any discomfort tends to disappear as both mother and baby establish the routine of breast-feeding.

Although breast is undoubtedly best, it is not always possible for a mother to breast-feed. Feeding problems such as mastitis, cracked nipples or an insufficient supply of milk do put many new mothers off the idea. Breast-feeding is also difficult while working, although expressed milk can be kept in bottles in the fridge and also freezes well. Mothers who experience problems will find their local branch of the National Childbirth Trust or La Leche League (a breast-feeding support network) both sympathetic and helpful. These organizations have experienced counsellors on call and can also arrange the hire of such useful equipment as electric breast pumps. For those who choose not to breast-feed, or who stop after the first few months, the next step is to choose a formula feed. Powdered milks are preferable to cow's milk because they are more easily digested and contain a more suitable ratio of nutrients for infants. Despite the glossy advertising campaigns, there is not much difference between the brands. As a leading paediatrician (who prefers to remain un-named) puts it: 'Do you really believe there is a difference between types of petrol? The same is true of baby milks. Your choice depends on who you want to give your money to.'

FIRST FOODS
Few babies should be given solids before the age of three

months and most should be having some by the age of six months: the majority of babies receive their first mouthfuls between the ages of four and six months. It is generally accepted that the longer you leave the introduction of solids the better. This is because the early introduction of certain foods is linked to allergy problems and food intolerances. The early use of cereal foods containing wheat gluten can predispose the baby to coeliac disease.

In America, some paediatricians suggest that solid foods are not given until a baby is six months old. However, it is important that all babies receive some solid food after this age as by then the iron reserves that they are born with will have run out. At the end of the day, no text-book knows the needs of each individual and ultimately, baby knows best. If a baby is hungry and fractious at three months, s/he may benefit from their first taste of something solid. If a baby is settled and thriving on milk alone, s/he may be fine until five or six months.

The first food any baby should be given is plain baby rice, mixed with a small amount of breast-milk or formula milk. This is the only food that should be given for the first fortnight of weaning. After two weeks, other foods may be introduced. Good first foods include mashed banana, puréed apple, carrot, parsnip and broccoli. Giving a baby a few mouthfuls of puréed fruits and vegetables is an ideal way of ensuring a steady supply of the ACE vitamins. Researchers have also noted that babies are more receptive to new tastes between the ages of six and eighteen months. By giving babies many different types of fresh fruits and vegetables we help to ensure that they will grow up willing to eat their greens.

Ideas about feeding babies are continually changing and the chances are that your mother fed you in a different way to the recommended guidelines today. For example, it is now suggested that you do not give cow's milk until a baby is a year old, and that formula follow-on milks should be given instead. This may help prevent any intolerance to cow's milk and provide more nutrients for the rapidly growing infant. Good nutrition from the earliest age is important and the Health Education Authority recommends giving a child supplementary vitamin drops until the age of two, and preferably until five years old. The Health Education Authority currently states: 'When babies start to drink normal cow's milk they should start receiving vitamin supplements, particularly vitamin D when there is too little exposure to sunlight to synthesis enough for the baby's needs.'

Vitamin drops are widely available from chemists and local health authority childcare clinics. The drops contain vitamins A (not beta-carotene), vitamin C and vitamin D. Cod-liver oil will supply vitamins A (again, not beta-caro-tene) and vitamin D. Cod liver oil should only be taken in-stead of vitamin drops, not at the same time, in case the baby receives too much of the retinol form of vitamin A. Orange-flavoured versions of cod liver oil are available and these also contain added vitamin C. Either vitamin drops or cod liver oil are a useful supplement for babies and toddlers but should not be their sole source of vita-mins. Small children will still need to eat fresh fruit and vegetables to obtain their valuable share of beta-carotene. They will also need to eat wholegrain bread and cereals for their vitamin E content.

The other main nutrient likely to be lacking in a baby's diet is iron. All babies are born with a good supply of iron and when this is added to the iron they automatically re-ceive from breast-milk or formula feeds the supply will last until they are five or six months old. After this time, babies need to be given foods containing iron, for example sieved green vegetables such as spinach or well-cooked eggs.

SUPPLEMENTS FOR BABIES
Optimum nutrition is important for all children and vita-min drops are available for all those on income support from the DSS. For babies on formula milk these drops are designed to top up the nutrients contained in the milk powder. The vitamin drops for babies and young children contain vitamin A 2000 IU, vitamin D 400 IU and vitamin C 50 mg. Children should not be given supplements

designed for adults as they may contain levels of some
nutrients that could be dangerous for a small child. There
are a few brands of multi-vitamins designed for small children, but these are not yet widely available. The best way
to ensure babies and toddlers receive their daily dose of
the ACE Plan vitamins is to make sure they eat plenty of
the ACE All-Star foods (see page 149).

BABY FOOD TIPS

- Avoid packets, bottles and jars where practical. Your
  baby will thrive on fresh foods that contain fewer 'fill-
  ers' such as modified starch or hydrolized vegetable
  protein. A sensible rule is to avoid anything labelled
  with ingredients that you don't understand.
- Keep it simple. A baby does not need fancy dishes, just
  plain, wholesome meals made with simple, fresh foods.
- Introduce new tastes one at a time. Aim to give your
  baby a new food two or three times a week. Good ones
  to try include sweet potato, broccoli, mango, kiwi and
  fresh pear.
- Some fruit and vegetables are nature's form of convenience foods when travelling. Un-zip a banana or slice a
  ripe pear in half and scoop out the insides with a spoon.
- If a food can be left raw, serve it this way to preserve its
  vitamins: for example, kiwi, avocado pear or paw paw.
- Ring the changes with different kinds of plain grains.
  Millet flakes, barley flakes, quinoa and oatmeal are all
  good baby foods. Serve plain, or add to a fruit or vegetable purée.
- Fruit juices are an ideal way to top up a baby's supplies
  of the ACE vitamins. Carrot juice is high in beta-carotene and is good to mix with baby rices. Apple juice is
  thought to be the easiest on an infant's stomach (dilute
  a small amount with pure water). Avoid baby drinks
  with added sugar as these have been shown to rot infant teeth (most now carry warnings on the label).
- Never add salt to a baby's food as it can damage the kid-
  neys. If you are giving a baby some of the family's food,
  make sure it isn't salted.

Childhood

The jury is still out on whether vitamins can improve a child's intelligence or not. Some studies suggest they do, a few have found that they do not. Studies have shown that children who were given vitamin supplements out-performed those who were given placebo pills. Those taking the vitamins showed an improvement equivalent of more than 4 IQ points, regardless of age, sex or original IQ of the child. Unfortunately, these results have not been repeated in subsequent trials and are now widely discredited. Regardless of whether vitamins boost brain power or not, there is no doubt that children need vitamins and minerals for their development. Parents have a fundamental duty to make sure their children receive the basic building-blocks for strong, healthy bodies.

Breakfast is a 'must-have' for all of us, but especially for children as it will keep their energy levels high and help them concentrate at school. Without breakfast, a child will suffer from a dip in energy at around 10-11 a.m. and is more likely to reach for a non-nutritious chocolate bar at breaktime. Breakfast is also a good time to ensure your children receive their vital dose of the ACE vitamins. Many cereals have added vitamins and minerals which can make a significant contribution to their daily intake. However, your choice of cereals should also be low in fat and sugar. Granola-style cereals may look healthy, but their fat content is often high. Likewise, all frosted sugar- or honey-coated cereals contain very high amounts of sugar. Choose plain cereals with no added sugar and opt for wholewheat varieties which will contain more vitamin E. In in doubt, check the nutrition panel on the side of each packet and compare notes on sugar, fat and salt content (the lower the better). You may well be surprised by the differences between brands. It's well worth getting into the habit of giving small children plain cereals so that they don't develop a sweet tooth and demand the frosted varieties. Breakfast cereals should be supplemented with fruit juice or a piece of fresh fruit, to give your child good levels of beta-carotene and vitamin C (see the vitamin content tables on pages 52 and 58). Fresh juices are better than squash or those made from concentrates as fewer of the antioxidant vitamins are lost in the production process. Whole grains in the form of wholemeal toast or porridge, which contain some vitamin E, are also good for filling up hungry kids. Breakfast is the meal that parents often find the easiest to control – so make sure your children fill up on the ACE vitamins before leaving the door.

SCHOOLDAYS

Any hopes of monitoring what our children eat tend to get abandoned as soon as they go to school. Although we can encourage them to make healthy choices, the influence of advertisers is often greater than parental persuasion. Children are highly susceptible to TV advertising and peer pressure. My two-year-old can't be the only one to demand a particular brand of yoghurt after seeing it advertised with a dancing hippo on television. What is advertised one morning invariably turns up in the lunchbox the next day. It is frankly horrifying to see what some children eat at school. A spot-check at one primary school in Coventry revealed at least half a dozen lunch-boxes packed only with chocolate bars and tins of cola. It is important to resist the temptation to give in to advertisers and peer pressure just for a bit of peace. It helps if you can leave the children at home while doing the supermarket shop for the week ahead. This way the trolley is less likely to be filled with high-fat, high-sugar, low-vitamin foods that cheat growing bodies of their optimum nutrition.

Don't use sweets for treats. It is easy to get hooked on sugar, especially if you grow up to think of it as a reward for good behaviour. Try substituting other things, such as exotic fruits rich in the ACE vitamins. If your children take packed lunches to school, make sure they are packed with goodness. By all means add the odd sweet snack or occasional packet of crisps, but it should be stressed that these are rare treats and not regular foods. The switch to healthier eating is simple to make and will dramatically boost vitamin levels. For example, wholemeal bread contains around ten times as much vitamin E as white bread. Carrot sticks are a reasonable source of beta-carotene, while tangarines and, to a lesser extent, apples, give good levels of vitamin C. At the end of the day, what goes into your children is fuelling their future. The choice is yours.

School dinners are a common cause of complaint countrywide. They are all too frequently either simply unavailable or unappetizing and left largely uneaten. Parents can help to encourage head teachers and catering managers by requesting a review of meal arrangements and menus. For example, baked potatoes contain far less fat than chips and provide more fibre and vitamin C. High-fat, sugar-filled puddings can be replaced with fresh fruit which is a natural source of the ACE vitamins. No one is saying it is easy to resist the temptation of colourful chocolate bars, lurid fizzy drinks and crunchy crisp packets – especially when they are so extensively advertised. However, some schools have successfully banned sweets altogether. Although it is difficult to convince them at first, children do settle down to accept that they can only snack on apples, grapes, bananas, dried fruit and nuts. This option is not only more nutritious, it can work out much cheaper too.

SUPPLEMENTS FOR CHILDREN

Children are more susceptible than adults to vitamin toxicity. The two most important vitamins to watch out for are vitamin A (retinol) and vitamin D. Large daily doses above vitamin A 4000 IU and vitamin D 400 IU are not recommended. If your children do not eat large amounts of fresh fruit and vegetables every day they may be falling short on the ACE vitamins. It is impossible to set hard and fast guidelines on the levels of these vitamins that should be supplemented, principally because research has not yet been carried out to establish the specific antioxidant needs of children. In any case, this will depend on lifestyle factors such as their diet and whether they live in a polluted area or breathe in cigarette smoke (both of which will increase their needs). Rather than laying down rigid rules, I would suggest that parents make up their own minds about the needs of their children, based on the evidence currently available. However, I should add that my own small children are encouraged to eat a diet naturally rich in the ACE vitamins and also receive a daily supplement of beta-carotene 10 mg, vitamin C 100 mg and 20 mg of natural vitamin E (30 IU).

LUNCH-BOX TIPS
Pack your child's lunch-box with good sources of the ACE vitamins.

- Wholemeal bread is one of the handiest sources of vitamin E. Make sure the label says 'wholemeal' as brown bread and granary loaves are not the same.
- Add salad vegetables to sandwiches to boost their vitamin content, for example, sliced tomatoes with cheese, green peppers with chicken and plenty of cress with egg mayonnaise.
- Pack plenty of fruit! Experiment with more adventurous ideas such as fruit kebabs made with exotic varieties.
- Cherry tomatoes are popular with kids and a good source of beta-carotene.
- Add a portion of pasta salad, made with extra peas, beans and tomatoes.
- Soup served from a wide-necked thermos flask is a great winter warmer for children. Home-made vegetable soup is a good option, otherwise add peas and beans to canned tomato soup for plenty of beta-carotene and vitamin C.
- Sticks of raw carrot are a beta-carotene booster. Add cottage cheese or houmus for dipping.
- Add wholemeal currant buns instead of iced cakes and biscuits. These have far less sugar and more vitamin E.
- Fruit yoghurts can be a good source of vitamins. Check the label to make sure there is more fruit than sugar! (The fruit content should be listed first).
- Fresh fruit is a must for all lunch-boxes. Oranges are the best source of vitamin C, tangerines and satsumas are good too and easier for small hands to peel.

- Make nutritious vitamin E-enriched snacks such as plain popcorn tossed with sunflower seeds and a dash of tamari or soya sauce.
- Nuts are also a good source of vitamin E. Add a handful of unsalted brazils, almonds or hazelnuts instead of sweets. Small children can choke on nuts, so give them nut-butter sandwiches instead. Most health food shops sell jars of almond and brazil nut butters as well as the more common peanut butter.

Adolescence

The teenage years are turbulent times. Not only does the body undergo rapid development, which can create a sense of insecurity, but these years are also filled with stresses such as exams and first love. It is ironic that at a time when teenagers most need the back-up of good nutrition, they are least likely to be achieving it. Every teenager has a different biological body-clock, but it is not unusual for an adolescent to grow 10 cm in height or add more than 5 kg in body weight in a year. These dramatic growth spurts need to be fuelled by the best forms of nutrition. Active adolescent boys may need up to 4000 calories a day (twice the normal adult man's recommended intake). Less active boys who spend more time playing with computer games or watching TV than playing sport obviously need fewer calories than this, as do teenage girls. But good nutrition means much more than filling up on high-calorie foods. Teenage bodies need high intakes of good-quality foods, such as nuts, a good source of protein and vitamin E, to ensure healthy muscle growth. Both boys and girls require good supplies of iron for the increased muscle development and blood supply. Foods rich in iron include dark green leafy vegetables, eggs, beans and lentils. Teenage girls may need extra iron supplements if they have heavy periods. Supplements are also very necessary for vegetarians, red meat being one of the best sources of iron.

FOOD FADS

As independence increases, teenagers tend to make their

own decisions concerning the foods they will eat. Fast-foods and convenient, ready-made meals frequently replace home cooking. Fresh fruit and vegetables often fail to pass the adolescent taste-test. As a result, teenagers tend to eat fewer of the ACE vitamins. Unfortunately, if these bad eating habits become entrenched, the health of future generations could be affected.

Other more encouraging eating habits acquired in teenage years can also follow through to adulthood. The number of those making the switch to vegetarianism is highest in the teenage age group. This could be because teenagers stop eating meat once they become aware of the cruelty issues, or they may simply consider it more trendy to be a vegetarian. When properly implemented, meat-free eating can be very healthy. Vegetarians tend to have lower cholesterol levels and lower blood pressure, making them less susceptible to heart disease. They are also known to have lower rates of cancer than meat eaters. However, this could also be attributed to eating more vegetables and whole grains that contain the ACE vitamins. Teenage vegetarians should be aware that they need to keep their protein and iron levels high, and eat plenty of beans, nuts and dark green leafy vegetables. Vegans, who do not eat any animal products such as milk or cheese, may need to take a supplement of vitamin B12 (commonly only found in meat and fortified yeast extract spreads) and should eat plenty of calcium-rich foods such as grains, nuts, seeds and green leafy vegetables.

The rise in food-related disorders during adolescence is extremely worrying. Most cases of eating disorders such as anorexia and bulimia make their first appearance at this time. Depriving the body of essential nutrients during a period of such intensive growth and development can lead to permanent weaknesses in later life. Dieting is also to be discouraged as it disturbs the body's natural metabolism and can lead to future health problems. Those worried about their weight should switch to low-fat foods such as yoghurt and skimmed milk that contain just as much calcium as the full-fat varieties, but with far fewer calories. All teenagers should eat the important energy or fuel foods at every meal and these include wholemeal bread, pasta, rice, cereals, pulses and potatoes. These will satisfy the hungriest appetites without piling on the pounds. Fruit and vegetables provide lots of essential vitamins and minerals too, including the ACE vitamins, so teenagers should aim to have at least four portions every day.

THINK BEFORE YOU DRINK
If you are old enough to drink, be wise enough not to. If you don't drink, don't start. However, most teenagers do experiment with alcohol during adolescence and can fall into the habit of regular drinking. You should be aware that drinking any kind of alcohol increases your chances of developing certain forms of cancer in later life. These include cancer of the breast, rectum and pancreas. If you drink large amounts of alcohol (especially if you smoke as well), you are also at much greater risk of contracting cancer of the mouth, oesophagus and larynx. In addition to the long-term cancer risk, there is also the short-term depletion of certain nutrients. Not only does alcohol interfere with the absorption of some vitamins, it can also reduce the appetite and make you more likely to skip meals. If you do drink, limit your consumption to less than one pure ounce of alcohol a day, roughly equivalent to two cans of beer or two small glasses of wine.

SUPPLEMENTS FOR TEENAGERS
In an ideal world, teenagers would eat a thoroughly healthy and perfectly balanced diet every day. We all know that this is rarely the case. There is peer pressure to choose fashionable foods and fast foods which are often not the most nutritious. A recent survey by the Department of Health revealed some worrying deficiencies in the foods eaten by adolescent girls, showing, for example, that about half of all teenager girls never, or only occasionally, drink milk. This is the most important source of calcium which is so vital for bone development during

periods of rapid growth. Many adolescent girls are also at risk of iron deficiency which causes anaemia. The survey found that at least 80 per cent of young teenager girls eat less than the RDA of iron, and are therefore at extra risk of deficiency due to their monthly blood loss. The Department of Health found further real evidence of vitamin deficiency as all the girls surveyed consumed less than the recommended daily allowances of vitamin B6 and vitamin D. Given this scenario, the only option for teenagers who refuse to eat healthily is to give them a vitamin and mineral supplement. This applies especially to the ACE vitamins which are mainly found in foods that teenagers most frequently avoid, such as fresh fruits, vegetables and whole grains. Deciding on the levels of these vitamins to be supplemented is a difficult question. The answer lies somewhere between the levels given to small children and adults, and depends to a large extent on what foods the adolescent is eating and where the deficiencies may lie. There are several brands of vitamin supplements created with teenagers in mind, but many of these contain vitamin A in the form of retinol, not beta-carotene. It is important to check the labels before you buy and make sure that the supplement lists beta-carotene, vitamin C and vitamin E among its ingredients.

TEENAGE TIPS
Growing bodies need to get the best from foods. Check out your nutrition needs:
- Do you eat lean red meat, dark green leafy vegetables, beans and lentils?

Answer no and you may need an iron supplement.
- Do you eat several servings of fresh fruit and vegetables every day?

Answer no and you may need a beta-carotene supplement.
- Do you eat oranges, tomatoes or drink fresh juices once or twice a day?

Answer no and you may need a vitamin C supplement.

- Do you eat wholemeal bread, wheatgerm or other whole grains every day?

Answer no and you may need a vitamin E supplement.

Adults

Despite the information about healthy living available, the vast majority of us continue with thoroughly unhealthy habits. A recent government report, compiled in 1993, paints a grim picture of an overweight population, reluctant to make any dramatic change in eating and drinking habits, slow to take any form of exercise and struggling to give up smoking. The survey of almost 3000 men and women found that a quarter had already suffered one serious illness linked to heart disease, such as angina, diabetes or high blood pressure. More than two-thirds had blood cholesterol levels above the optimum limit, and the number of obese men had almost doubled in the last seven years. Despite this shocking state of affairs, three-quarters of those surveyed maintained that their general health was 'good' or even 'very good'. However, the Chief Medical Officer, Dr Kenneth Calman, is urging every one of us to adopt healthier changes in our lifestyle.

Eating habits are hard to change once we reach adulthood as our likes and dislikes are firmly established during childhood and teenage years. Hopefully, by the time we are fully grown we have developed a taste for the healthier foods, such as fresh fruits and vegetables. Eating more fruits and vegetables is such an easy, convenient and relatively cheap option that it is hard to understand why it should be a problem. But the very idea of eating a well-balanced diet is far from a reality for some. For example, Scottish shoppers spend more on tobacco and alcohol than they do on fruit and vegetables. In Scotland, a third of all men and a fifth of all women do not eat enough fresh produce to supply their daily needs. This failure to have a well-balanced diet could be an important clue as to why Scotland tops the European list for deaths due to heart disease.

Healthy eating takes on more significance as we grow

older and the main life-threatening diseases loom on the horizon. Few of us consider the state of our arteries while we are young, but become increasingly conscious of our internal health as time goes by. The principal diseases that cause death in Britain are coronary heart disease (including circulatory disorders such as strokes) and cancer. As we have seen in the previous chapter, these may be heavily influenced by the amounts of ACE vitamins in our diet. Therefore it makes sense to eat plenty of foods containing antioxidant nutrients, such as green leafy vegetables and citrus fruits, throughout our adult life. The American Cancer Society recommends eating five to nine portions (each measuring 1 teacup) of fruit and vegetables daily as a preventive measure against cancer. There can be no doubt that the Western diet eaten by all developed countries is the least healthy. The scientific community at large agrees that we must all dramatically increase our intake of whole grains, fruits and vegetables which are not only high in dietary fibre, and low in fat and refined sugar, but are also our best sources of the ACE vitamins.

THE ACE PLAN EATING PYRAMID

The ACE Plan eating pyramid is an at-a-glance guide to a healthier diet. At the base of the pyramid are starchy foods, such as bread and potatoes, which form the foundation of healthy eating. Aim to eat five to nine portions a day. Next come the fruits and vegetables which also provide plenty of fibre as well as the important ACE vitamins. Aim to eat five to nine portions a day. Protein should be eaten occasionally, and women should especially focus on their calcium intake from dairy products. Oils and fats should be used sparingly, and sugar should be avoided.

PYRAMID PORTIONS
- protein:
    one portion = 3 oz/75 g lean meat or fish
    2 eggs
    10 oz/300 g cooked beans or lentils

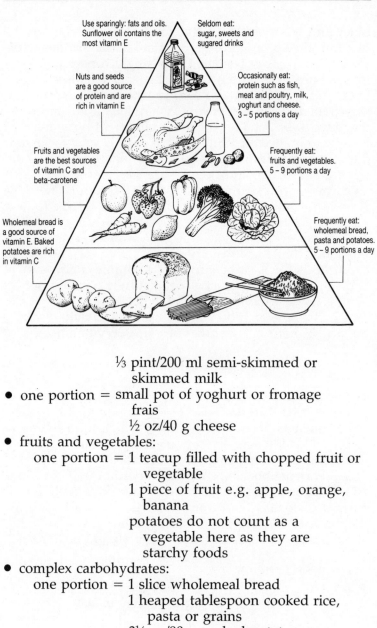

$\frac{1}{3}$ pint/200 ml semi-skimmed or skimmed milk

- one portion = small pot of yoghurt or fromage frais

  $\frac{1}{2}$ oz/40 g cheese

- fruits and vegetables:

  one portion = 1 teacup filled with chopped fruit or vegetable

  1 piece of fruit e.g. apple, orange, banana

  potatoes do not count as a vegetable here as they are starchy foods

- complex carbohydrates:

  one portion = 1 slice wholemeal bread

  1 heaped tablespoon cooked rice, pasta or grains

  $3\frac{1}{2}$ oz/90 g cooked potatoes

ACE ALL-STARS

- Top for beta-carotene: carrots, broccoli, tomatoes, spinach, cantaloupe melon, mango, apricots
- Top for vitamin C: oranges, blackcurrants, strawberries, green peppers, kale, Brussels sprouts, tomatoes
- Top for vitamin E: avocado, sunflower seeds, sunflower oil, whole grains, soya beans
- Top for selenium: bran, wheatgerm, tuna, onions, garlic, mushrooms

The ACE vitamins are present in almost all fruits and vegetables, although some contain far more than others. The amount of ACE vitamins that actually ends up on our plates depends to a large extent on storing, preparation and cooking. Lightly cooked – steamed or microwaved – vegetables preserve greater levels of vitamins than if they are boiled until mushy. However, the trend for pre-peeled and sliced vegetables and for storage under strong shop lights means that we end up with less beta-carotene and vitamin C. Orange juice is one of the best sources of vitamin C, yet its levels start to decline the moment it is put on the open shelf.

SUPPLEMENTS FOR ADULTS

Vitamins and minerals are widely present in many foods, so why should the average healthy adult take a supplement? The answer is that even the most well-balanced diet is likely to fall short of our antioxidant requirements today. Vitamin supplements are no substitute for a healthy diet, but taking them regularly is an ideal way to guarantee that your needs are being met at all times.

There is a growing lobby of scientific opinion to support taking a daily supplement of certain nutrients. Modern life requires an antidote to the persistent air pollution, smoking and drinking that destroy the normal functioning of some vitamins. The argument for supplements is further strengthened when we look at the losses of vitamins and minerals due to cooking, storage, food processing and the condition of the soil in which crops are grown. In addition, the results of many surveys around the world show that high levels of the ACE vitamins result in low levels of several widespread and serious diseases.

● Beta-carotene
Government figures show that the average daily intake of beta-carotene is about 2 mg. Other studies show that the lowest levels of beta-carotene are among young adults and that women aged between sixteen and twenty-four eat on average only 1.6 mg of beta-carotene a day, although this rises to 2.4 mg and 2.8 mg respectively among fifty- to sixty-four-year-olds. These figures are worryingly low, particularly in relation to beta-carotene intake in the young. As we have seen, brightly coloured fruits and vegetables are the best sources, but even these can vary. For example, Savoy cabbage contains 0.3 mg per 100 g serving, while spring cabbage has 0.5 mg per 100 g serving – a difference of 60 per cent. Either way, you will have to eat a great deal of cabbage to obtain correct levels of beta-carotene. According to Professor Diplock, the optimum daily intake of beta-carotene may be around 12-15 mg. It would be difficult, he says, to achieve these levels even by eating a diet containing large amounts of fresh fruit and vegetables, so taking a beta-carotene supplement may be the only way to achieve these levels of intake.

● Vitamin C
In theory, vitamin C is one of the easiest nutrients for us to obtain from our food as it is widely available in many fruits and vegetables, including oranges, blackcurrants, strawberries, Brussels sprouts and potatoes. However, the body has limited storage facilities for vitamin C, so we need to top up our supplies regularly throughout the day. This means frequently eating or drinking something that will provide a good quantity of vitamin C. A vitamin C supplement is the only other option. Our vitamin C levels are not only influenced by what we eat, there are several other factors that can deplete our supplies. Levels are lowered by smoking (including passive smoking), heavy drinking

and taking medicinal drugs including aspirin, antibiotics and corticosteroids. Women who take the contraceptive pill are also likely to have lower levels of vitamin C as the synthetic oestrogens reduce the amount available in the bloodstream. Vitamin C is also reduced by air pollution and by drinking tea and coffee. So if we finish our meal with a cup of coffee we are automatically reducing the amount of vitamin C we have just eaten. These factors all lead to the conclusion that we are likely to need a daily supplement. According to Professor Diplock, the suggested optimum intake of vitamin C is 100-150 mg every day. Some nutritionists advocate taking even higher doses, especially to combat the effects of pollution. Other scientists specializing in vitamin C research maintain that the ideal daily intake seems to be in the range of 50-500 mg, depending on state of health, age and social habits such as smoking. Those who smoke may need an additional 60-70 mg per day.

• Vitamin E

Our need for vitamin E directly relates to the amount of polyunsaturated fats we eat. High levels of polyunsaturated fats eaten in the diet increases our need for it and prevents these fats from turning rancid within the body. Nature provides foods that are high in fat with their own supplies of vitamin E – nuts, olives and sunflower seeds (all high in vegetable fat) are also excellent sources. However, the problems arise when food-processing techniques strip away levels of vitamin E in these foods. Many manufacturers extract the vitamin E and other nutrients from vegetable oils from olives, sunflower seeds and soya beans, to leave a clear, bland oil for bottling. This means that if we use these oils for cooking our cells are not receiving the protection they need from vitamin E. Instead, many oil refiners sell the vitamin E on to the food supplement industry, and we must buy it back in the form of supplements. All vegetable oils or oil-based foods such as sunflower spread, should contain vitamin E. If in doubt, question the manufacturer. Unrefined and cold-pressed vegetable oils have more vitamin E than highly refined cooking oils. If you are using a highly refined cooking oil, you would be well advised to take an additional vitamin E supplement. Even if you do eat a diet high in foods containing vitamin E, you are only likely to be consuming around 20 mg (30 IU) a day. According to Professor Diplock, the optimum daily intake of vitamin E is 50-80 mg (75-120 IU). The many studies in the UK and USA on disease prevention are generally based on much larger amounts of up to 800 IU of vitamin E every day.

TOP TIPS FOR ACE EATERS
- Side salads are a good way of eating extra vitamins, but make sure they contain the right ingredients. Pale lettuce and cucumber contain few vitamins. The best salad veggies are red and green peppers, watercress, tomatoes and carrots.
- Potatoes are a good source of vitamin C, but it does depend on how you cook them. A baked jacket potato is the best option. Mass-produced spuds that have been peeled, chopped and left soaking in water contain much less vitamin C.
- Buy fresh and eat it fresh! Fruit and vegetables have a limited lifespan, so store them in a cool, dark place and eat soon after purchase.
- Wash fruit thoroughly before eating, but avoid peeling. The highest concentrations of beta-carotene are found in the skin.
- Make more use of fruit – serve cantaloupe melon and strawberries as a starter, make chilled fruit soups, fresh fruit purées for desserts, unusual combinations in fruit salads and fruit bowls.
- Herbs are an excellent source of vitamin C. Sprinkle freshly chopped parsley on to soups, salads and vegetable dishes.
- Eat more vegetables raw, such as crunchy cauliflower florets, courgette sticks and shredded raw cabbage. However, we actually absorb more beta-carotene from carrots when they have been lightly cooked.

- Frozen vegetables are a good alternative to fresh and may even contain more vitamins. For example, peas and beans are picked and frozen immediately which means they can have more nutrients than a piece of elderly broccoli lurking at the bottom of the fridge.
- Be guided by colour: red, yellow and orange fruits and vegetables are all good sources of beta-carotene. Good examples include mango, apricots, carrots and red peppers. Dark green vegetables such as spinach, broccoli and Brussels sprouts are also a good source of beta-carotene, vitamins C and E.
- Ideally steam or microwave vegetables. If you boil them, add them to a pan of shallow boiling water. This helps speed cooking time and prevent vitamin losses.
- Vegetables should be eaten as soon as they are cooked. Discard the hot-plate or hostess trolley in favour of serving vegetables straight from the pan. Don't keep meals warm in the oven, try and batch-cook if people are eating at different times.
- Nuts and seeds are the easiest source of vitamin E to snack on, but they should be vacuum-sealed to delay rancidity. Once bought, store in a cool, dark place and eat quickly.
- Cooking oils should be stored in a cool, dark place to prevent rancidity. Adding the contents of a vitamin E capsule will help prevent the oil from going off.
- Invest in a larger fridge to store all fresh fruits, vegetables, nuts, seeds and cooking oils. This will keep your foods not only cool, but also in the dark.
- Smoked foods produce nitrosamines in the stomach which are linked to cancer. Fortunately, both vitamin C and vitamin E prevent their formation, so squeeze lemon juice on to smoked salmon and eat smoked meats such as salami with a dab of sunflower oil mayonnaise.

THE ACE CROP CALENDAR
Seasonal good buys make nutritional and financial good sense. No only are seasonal crops cheaper, they are also

less likely to have sat in cold storage for several months, which reduces their vitamin levels. Many imported fruit and vegetables, such as avocados, kiwi fruits and bananas, are now good buys all year round.

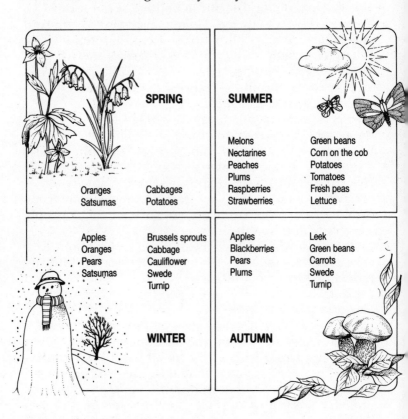

SPRING

Oranges	Cabbages
Satsumas	Potatoes

SUMMER

Melons	Green beans
Nectarines	Corn on the cob
Peaches	Potatoes
Plums	Tomatoes
Raspberries	Fresh peas
Strawberries	Lettuce

WINTER

Apples	Brussels sprouts
Oranges	Cabbage
Pears	Cauliflower
Satsumas	Swede
	Turnip

AUTUMN

Apples	Leek
Blackberries	Green beans
Pears	Carrots
Plums	Swede
	Turnip

The ACE Way to Weight-loss

In Britain, most women watch their weight and the vast majority follow some kind of restricted diet at some point in their lives. But being fat is by no means only a female affliction. The latest figures from the 1993 Health of the Nation document show that the number of seriously over-weight men has doubled in the last seven years. The only way to lose weight is to cut calories and increase exercise.

Many women struggle to keep their weight down and become obsessed with losing just a few pounds. When talking about weight loss and slimming it is important to put this into perspective: being grossly overweight is a health hazard. It can contribute to heart disease and diabetes, and will also put a great deal of strain on the joints. This makes it increasingly difficult to get around and increases the chances of developing further problems such as varicose veins. Obesity is at the extreme end of weight gain and middle-aged women are most often affected. Those who are fat cannot be as healthy as those who are nearer their ideal bodyweight (see chart below). However, being under-weight is not healthy either. Fashion magazines and advertisers do women no favours by portraying pin-thin models as the ideal female form. Most models are born either genetically skinny or half-starve themselves to stay thin.

Unfortunately, cutting down on calories can also dramatically decrease our levels of important nutrients, which may lead to health problems. For example, women need to keep their reserves of calcium high in order to maintain bone density and help prevent osteoporosis (thinning of the bones). The best sources of calcium are dairy products like milk and cheese, green leafy vegetables including broccoli, and sunflower seeds. Iron is another important nutrient for all menstruating women who lose some of their iron supply in their monthly period. Supplies of the ACE vitamins should be kept high by eating plenty of fresh fruits, vegetables and whole grains. Fortunately, these foods are also the slimmer's best friends as they are low in fat and high in goodness.

As anyone caught in the 'yo-yo' pattern of losing and gaining weight will know, very low-calorie diets only offer short-term weight loss. This is because they slow down the metabolism as the body shuts down its systems to preserve as much energy as possible. After a while, the body simply learns to get by on less fuel. This means that as soon as you resume normal eating habits and eat your previous levels of calories, the weight piles back on. Worst of all, these pounds become even more difficult to lose. There is no quick, short-cut to weight loss. The only sensible answer is long-term slimming, eating fewer high-fat, high-sugar foods and choosing more of the ACE All-Stars (see page 149). Regular exercise is also important to keep the metabolism high and burn off extra calories.

Eating a low-fat diet is one of the best ways to reduce calories and stay slim. Many low-fat diets advise avoiding high-fat foods such as nuts, avocado pears and vegetable oils, but these are also our best sources of vitamin E.

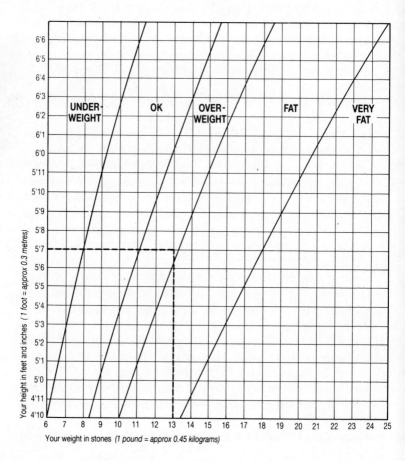

Fortunately, however, these vegetable fats contain mono-unsaturated oils which are healthier than the saturated fats found in animal produce. So, although high in calories, they will not clog our arteries as saturated fat does, and it is advisable to eat small quantities of these foods for overall health. For those who are determined to count every calorie and avoid these foods altogether, a supplement of vitamin E is an alternative. Each capsule of vitamin E contains only approximately 5 calories, yet provides the body with far more vitamin E than is found in a portion of avocado pear or brazil nuts.

ACE SLIMMING TIPS

- Fill up on starchy foods such as bread, pasta, noodles, rice, potatoes, sweet potatoes, chapattis and dishes made from maize, millet and cornmeal. These contain fewer calories than high-fat, sugary goods. Wholemeal bread contains vitamin E and plenty of fibre to fill you up.
- Eat fewer high-fat foods and cut down on cakes, biscuits and pastries (all are surprisingly high in fat). Use low-fat yoghurt or fromage frais (labelled less than 1 per cent fat) instead of cream or evaporated milk. Try half-fat cheese and cottage cheese as lower-fat alternatives.
- Switch to semi-skimmed milk which tastes like full-fat milk but has had the cream removed. Skimmed milk is lower still in fat but has a 'thinner' taste which can take some getting used to.
- Salads are good for slimmers and many salad ingredients, such as carrots, watercress and tomatoes, are an excellent source of beta-carotene. Make salad dressings with a dash of olive oil (a good source of vitamin E), low-fat yoghurt and lemon juice (rich in vitamin C). Use this instead of mayonnaise or salad cream.
- Boost your levels of beta-carotene and you will automatically be eating a lower-fat diet. Increase your fruit and vegetable rations to *at least* five generous portions per day. This will also help fill you up and reduce the temptation of sweets or high-fat snacks.

- Buy the leanest cuts of meats possible and trim off all visible fat. Don't eat the skin from chicken or turkey as this is high in fat.
- When cooking foods, grill, steam or microwave to preserve their nutrient content. Avoid over-cooking vegetables. Keep the calories down by not frying foods.
- Fresh fruit juices are a good source of vitamin C. Try diluting fresh orange, grapefruit or pineapple juice with sparkling water for a low-calorie spritzer.
- Tinned fruits are also a handy source of vitamins. Choose varieties packed in natural juice, not sugar syrup.
- If you are avoiding certain foods high in vegetable fats, including nuts, seeds, avocados and cooking oil, you are probably falling short of your daily vitamin E requirement. Consider taking a daily supplement.

Pregnancy

The nine months of pregnancy make unique demands on the body. Not only does a pregnant woman have to feed herself, she is also providing the nourishment for another growing human being. Not surprisingly, this is an especially important time to keep nutrient levels high. It is during the first three months of pregnancy that all the organs of the baby are fully formed, making optimum nutrition essential. Unfortunately, the first trimester is also when you are most likely to be suffering from morning sickness or feel too tired to eat properly. If you suspect you may not be eating enough of the right nutrients, vitamin and mineral supplements can be very helpful. All pregnant women are currently advised by the government to take folic acid supplements to reduce the likelihood of spina bifida affecting the baby. Many are also advised by their doctors to take an iron supplement to prevent anaemia, which in a mild form may be present in one in three pregnant women: the symptoms include pallor, tiredness and lethargy. Most pregnant women feel tired, especially during the last few months, another reason why it is important to avoid running short of iron.

ACE PREGNANCY TIPS

- Snack on fresh fruit to help prevent morning sickness and boost vitamin levels.
- Eat smaller, more frequent meals to keep energy reserves high.
- Make sure each meal includes at least two portions of fruit or vegetables. This will help to ensure you receive a steady supply of beta-carotene and vitamin C.
- Whole grains help prevent constipation and piles (common in pregnancy) and are also a good source of vitamin E. Try to eat at least three servings daily.
- Eat plenty of dairy products such as low-fat yoghurt and cottage cheese to provide the baby with the calcium needed for strong teeth and bones. Fish with edible bones, such as sardines, are also a good source of calcium.
- Vitamin D is needed to absorb calcium. The best sources are fortified margarines and oily fish such as sardines and mackerel. Vitamin D is also made in the skin from sunlight, so try to get out for a while every day.
- Good sources of iron include green leafy vegetables, lean red meat, dried fruits and nuts.
- Take a folic acid supplement from the time of conception through the first three months of pregnancy to help prevent neural tube birth defects.
- Consider taking a vitamin E supplement in the last three months of pregnancy as this is when the vitamin is passed on to the baby.
- Avoid drinking alcohol as it passes across the placental barrier and may damage the foetus.
- Don't smoke. Not only do smokers have low birth-weight babies but there is a possibility that smoking affects the child's mental development in later life. Smoking also depletes vitamin C, which is especially necessary during pregnancy to build a strong immune system for the baby.
- Vitamin A is an important nutrient during pregnancy, but avoid supplements containing high levels of retinol.

Large doses of synthetic retinol have been linked to birth defects in the USA. For this reason, it is wise to switch to beta-carotene which the body converts to vitamin A as needed.

- Rubbing a vitamin-E enriched cream into the skin may help prevent stretch marks after the birth. If stretch marks appear they may be slightly faded by the topical application of vitamin E (pierce the contents of a capsule and rub this into the mark night and morning). Vitamin E can also help fade Caesarian scars and studies show that it improves wound healing. Apply after the stitches have dissolved or been removed.

Age Concern

Elderly people are more likely to suffer from poor nutrition than the rest of the population. This may be due to low income, illness, loss of appetite, or mental or physical lethargy in meal preparation. Many old people living on their own simply don't bother to cook meals for one and live on an assortment of processed foods. The elderly are also likely to indulge a sweet tooth and many eat large amounts of fat-filled, sugary foods such as cakes and pastries. They may not be very mobile and unable to carry home heavy groceries such as fresh fruit and vegetables. In addition, the appetite decreases with age and inactivity, so more nutrients need to be packed into fewer foods. This is why it is so important for elderly people to eat foods that are especially nutritious. Many elderly people have limited knowledge of the new nutritional data on foods: for example, they may not be aware that although bread and cakes are easy to digest, they contain little in the way of vitamins.

The elderly are more likely to spend time indoors and may even be housebound. In this case, they are not receiving any vitamin D which is made in the skin by moderate exposure to sunlight. A vitamin D supplement is a good idea for any elderly person who does not go outdoors very often. Some studies show that the elderly are also likely to be low in vitamin C and folic acid (one of the B-complex vitamins). Research suggests that the majority of elderly people in Britain could have dangerously low levels of the ACE vitamins. Dr Tom Sanders, Reader in Nutrition at King's College, University of London, measured vitamin E and beta-carotene levels in sixty-five people over the age of seventy. He discovered that a staggering 90 per cent had levels that were below normal. According to Dr Sanders, 'The levels were really very low, suggesting these people are not receiving the protective effect afforded by these vitamins on certain diseases.'

There are many reasons why vitamin levels are lower in the elderly. For example, they may eat less fresh fruit because of the difficulty in peeling fruit such as oranges. They may also eat fewer fruits and vegetables because of difficulties in chewing. The elderly in institutions are particularly prone to a low intake of vitamin C because it is hard to maintain high levels in bulk-cooked food. Overcooked or puréed vegetables may be easier to digest, but the amounts of vitamins available are depleted. An Italian study in 1990 assessed the vitamin C status of sixty-four elderly women living in care compared to sixty-five women who lived at home. All the women lived in Rome and were aged from sixty to ninety. On average, those living at home had at least a third more vitamin C in their bloodstream than those in residential care. Of those with the lowest levels of vitamin C, many showed visible signs of vitamin C deficiency, including weakened hair and nails, swollen and bleeding gums and haemorrhaging skin spots. In these circumstances, a regular glass of fresh orange juice or simple daily supplement of vitamin C would make all the difference.

As we saw in the previous chapter, the ACE vitamins may be able to reduce the rise in certain cancers, a common killer amongst the elderly. According to Professor Blumberg at the Human Nutrition Research Centre at Tufts University, Boston, 'We have the evidence that shows high levels of antioxidants may inhibit lesions and even influence the regression of lesions.' The only way to achieve these high levels is by taking supplements. This is especially relevant for the elderly who tend to have poor appetites and eat frugally.

SUPPLEMENTS FOR THE ELDERLY

There is no doubt that the ACE vitamins play an important role in degenerative disease. This is why it is so important for the elderly to receive their fair share. Unfortunately, this age group is at risk of low levels of ACE vitamins due to poor diet and low appetite and a daily supplement would seem to be a sensible precaution. High levels of beta-carotene are likely to be lacking in old age, as the elderly move away from eating large amounts of fruits and vegetables, and a daily supplement of 15-25 mg is recommended. The government RDA for vitamin C for the elderly is currently 150 mg daily. For those who smoke this amount should be increased by around 75 mg, bringing the total to 225 mg a day. It is unlikely that the elderly regularly achieve this level through diet alone. Those who fall below this level should be increasing their intake of vitamin C-rich foods such as oranges, or taking a supplement. When it comes to vitamin E, the elderly are likely to obtain only low levels from food because good sources of vitamin E such as nuts and seeds are awkward to chew and difficult to digest. Other vitamin E-rich foods, such as asparagus and avocado, are expensive for those on pensions and may be unappealing. In this case, a supplement of vitamin E is the only way to achieve the levels of 50-80 mg (75-120 IU) recommended as our ideal daily intake.

ACE PLAN TRIVIA

Test your nutritional knowledge and be an ACE winner!

1. What does beta-carotene do in the body?
   (A: It works as an antioxidant as well as topping up levels of vitamin A.)

2. How can you tell if fruits and vegetables contain beta-carotene?
   (A: They are brightly coloured, e.g. carrots, tomatoes and spinach.)

3. By what other name is vitamin C known?
   (A: Ascorbic acid.)

4. What are the best food sources of vitamin E?
   (A: Vegetable oils, nuts, seeds, wholemeal flour, wheatgerm, avocados.)

5. Which has more vitamin C, apple juice or orange juice?
   (A: Fresh orange juice.)

6. Do smokers need more or less vitamin C?
   (A: Around 75 mg more vitamin C a day.)

7. Where does the vitamin E contained in capsules come from?
   (A: Vegetable oils such as soya bean or wheatgerm oil.)

8. Is synthetic or natural beta-carotene better absorbed by the body?
   (A: The natural form of beta-carotene is better absorbed.)

9. How can you tell if the natural form of vitamin E is in a supplement?
   (A: The label states 'natural-source vitamin E' or it is listed as d-alpha not dl-alpha.)

10. By what term are beta-carotene, vitamin C and vitamin E also known?
    (A: They are all antioxidants.)

Vitamin E Ready-reckoner

1.49 IU = 1 mg natural vitamin E
1 IU   = 0.67 mg vitamin E
25 IU   = 17 mg
50 IU   = 33.5 mg
100 IU = 67 mg
200 IU = 134 mg
300 IU = 201 mg
400 IU = 268 mg
500 IU = 335 mg
600 IU = 402 mg
700 IU = 469 mg
800 IU = 536 mg

The above table shows the values for d-alpha-tocopherol, the most potent form of natural source vitamin E.

Natural vitamin E
(in order of potency)
d-alpha-tocopherol
d-alpha-tocopheryl acetate
d-alpha-tocopheryl acid succinate

Synthetic vitamin E
(in order of potency)
dl-alpha-tocopherol
dl-alpha-tocopheryl acetate
dl-alpha-tocopheryl acid succinate

GLOSSARY

Alzheimer's disease
The progressive deterioration of the brain with subsequent loss of memory. Recognized as a mental disorder associated with ageing.

Antioxidant
A substance that prevents oxidation. Nutrients with antioxidant activity include beta-carotene, vitamin C and vitamin E.

Ascorbic acid
Another name for vitamin C.

Atherosclerosis
Damage to the main arteries due to a build-up of fatty deposits, especially cholesterol, that leads to heart disease.

Beta-carotene
A powerful antioxidant, unlike vitamin A which can be made from it. The main sources of beta-carotene in our foods our brightly coloured fruits and vegetables, such as carrots, apricots, spinach and broccoli.

Carotenoids
A group of plant pigments ranging in colour from yellow to red. There are over 650 naturally-occurring carotenoids, many of which have antioxidant properties. However, beta-carotene is one of the most active.

Cataract
The clouding of the lens in the eye associated with ageing. Studies indicate that the antioxidant vitamins may help prevent this.

Cell membrane
The double layer of fatty material and proteins that surrounds each living cell of all organisms.

Cholesterol
A fatty substance that has many important functions throughout the body. Excess cholesterol may be deposited in the artery lining.

Degenerative disease
The loss of the capacity of cells, tissues and organs needed for the body to function normally.

DNA
Deoxyribonucleic acid, the basic material in the chromosomes of each cell containing the genetic code of life.

Enzyme
A substance produced by the body that regulates biochemical reactions.

Free radical
A reactive particle that contains one or more unpaired electrons, causing it to be highly unstable and sometimes destructive within the body. Free radicals are encouraged by exposure to pollutants such as cigarette smoke. They age cells by damaging their structure and DNA.

HDL
Abbreviation for high-density lipoproteins, the vehicles that transport excess cholesterol away from the arteries and return it to the liver for disposal.

Hydrogenation
A biological and commercial process that turns oils into hard fats.

LDL
Abbreviation for low-density lipoproteins, the vehicles that carry fats around the body in the bloodstream. They are considered to be the 'bad' form of cholesterol as an excess can build up in the arteries and lead to atherosclerosis.

Lipid
A technical name for any type of fat, oil or other fatty substance.

Mitochondria
Small, rod-like parts of the cell that contain DNA.

Molecules
Organized groups of two or more atoms.

Oxidation
The process of using oxygen to release energy from cells. Its side-effect is to produce free radicals.

Ozone
A form of oxygen in which three atoms of the element combine to form the molecule O3. Ozone is a powerful oxidant and can produce free radicals when inhaled.

Placebo
A 'dummy' pill given to volunteers taking part in a blind clinical trial, in which participants do not know whether they are being given the active substance being tested or a placebo.

Polyunsaturates
A fatty acid that contains several double bonds between carbon atoms in its chain.

Protein
A family of molecules made by linking amino-acids together.

PUFA
Abbreviation for polyunsaturated fatty acid.

RDA
Abbreviation for Recommended Daily Allowance, the amount of vitamins and minerals 'needed to satisfy the needs of the population', as advised by governments.

Retinol
The active component of vitamin A.

Singlet oxygen
An active form of oxygen that can lead to free radical formation.

Superoxide dismutase
Otherwise known as SOD. An antioxidant enzyme found naturally in cells within the body. One form of the enzyme contains manganese and the other contains copper and zinc. It is important to fight free radicals.

Tocopherols
Forms of vitamin E. Natural vitamin E is labelled as d-alpha-tocopherol.

Trans-fats
Fatty acid that has hydrogen and carbon atoms in a double bond on the opposite sides of its normal chain.

Vitamins
Over a dozen essential nutrients that the body cannot make from other substances and which must therefore be supplied in the diet.

Vitamin A
The active component is retinol or retinyl palmitate.

Vitamin C
Otherwise known as l-ascorbic acid. This water-soluble substance is thought to be the most important antioxidant in cell fluids. Good sources include citrus fruits, tomatoes, cabbage and strawberries.

Vitamin E
Otherwise known as d-alpha tocopherol, which is the natural form, or dl-alpha tocopherol, which is the less effective synthetic version. Vitamin E is fat-soluble and is found in all cellular membranes. The best food sources are vegetable cooking oils and wheatgerm. We probably do not get enough vitamin E from our food and may benefit from taking a supplement.

Your Score

Section 1: Pollution

Q.1
Q.2
Q.3
Q.4
Q.5

Section 2: Smoking
Q.6
Q.7
Q.8
Q.9

Section 3: Radiation

Q.10
Q.11
Q.12
Q.13
Q.14
Q.15
Q.16
Q.17

Section 4: Alcohol

Q.18
Q.19
Q.20
Q.21

Your Score

Section 5: Diet

Q.22
Q.23
Q.24
Q.25
Q.26
Q.27
Q.28

Section 6: Exercise
Q.29
Q.30
Q.31

Section 7: Genetics

Q.32
Q.33
Q.34

Total Score [   ]

Score Sheet 2

Section 1: Pollution

Q.1
Q.2
Q.3
Q.4
Q.5

Section 2: Smoking
Q.6
Q.7
Q.8
Q.9

Section 3: Radiation

Q.10
Q.11
Q.12
Q.13
Q.14
Q.15
Q.16
Q.17

Section 4: Alcohol

Q.18
Q.19
Q.20
Q.21

Score Sheet 2

Section 5: Diet

Q.22
Q.23
Q.24
Q.25
Q.26
Q.27
Q.28

Section 6: Exercise
Q.29
Q.30
Q.31

Section 7: Genetics

Q.32
Q.33
Q.34

Total Score [   ]

Score Sheet 3

Section 1: Pollution

Q.1
Q.2
Q.3
Q.4
Q.5

Section 2: Smoking
Q.6
Q.7
Q.8
Q.9

Section 3: Radiation

Q.10
Q.11
Q.12
Q.13
Q.14
Q.15
Q.16
Q.17

Section 4: Alcohol

Q.18
Q.19
Q.20
Q.21

Score Sheet 3

Section 5: Diet

Q.22
Q.23
Q.24
Q.25
Q.26
Q.27
Q.28

Section 6: Exercise
Q.29
Q.30
Q.31

Section 7: Genetics

Q.32
Q.33
Q.34

Total Score [   ]

If you would like to find out more about the ACE way of eating, watch out for *The ACE Plan Weight-Loss for Life* by Liz Earle. Packed with tips for lifelong healthy eating, the book contains tasty ACE recipes the whole family will enjoy. *The ACE Plan Weight-Loss for Life* will be available from all good bookshops from February 1994.